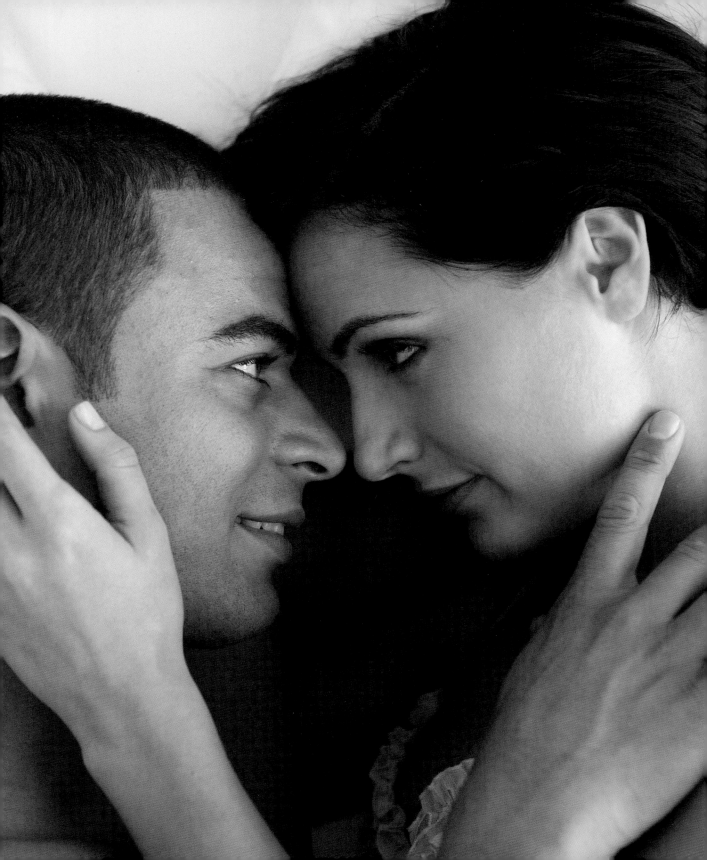

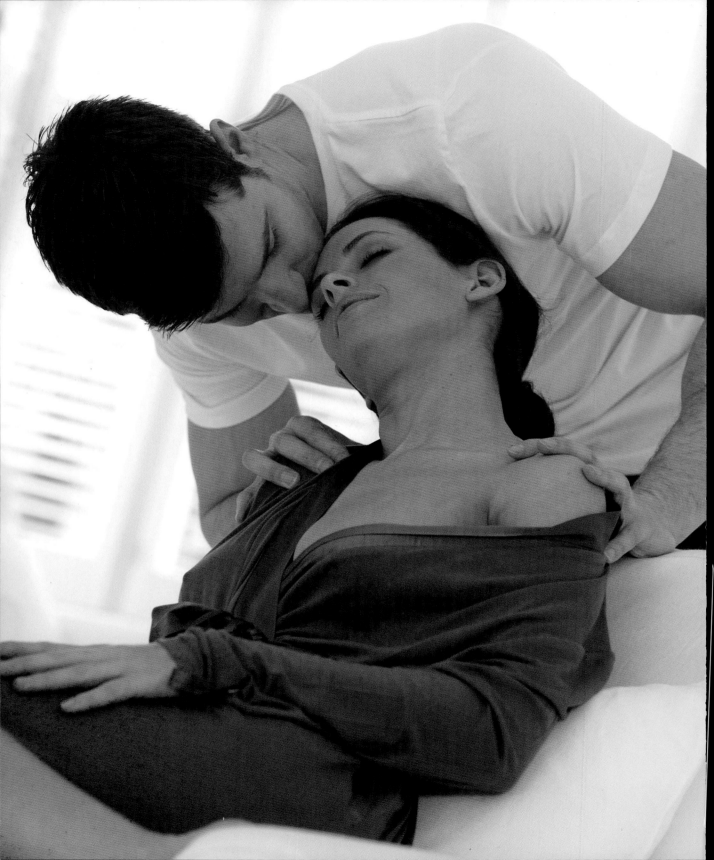

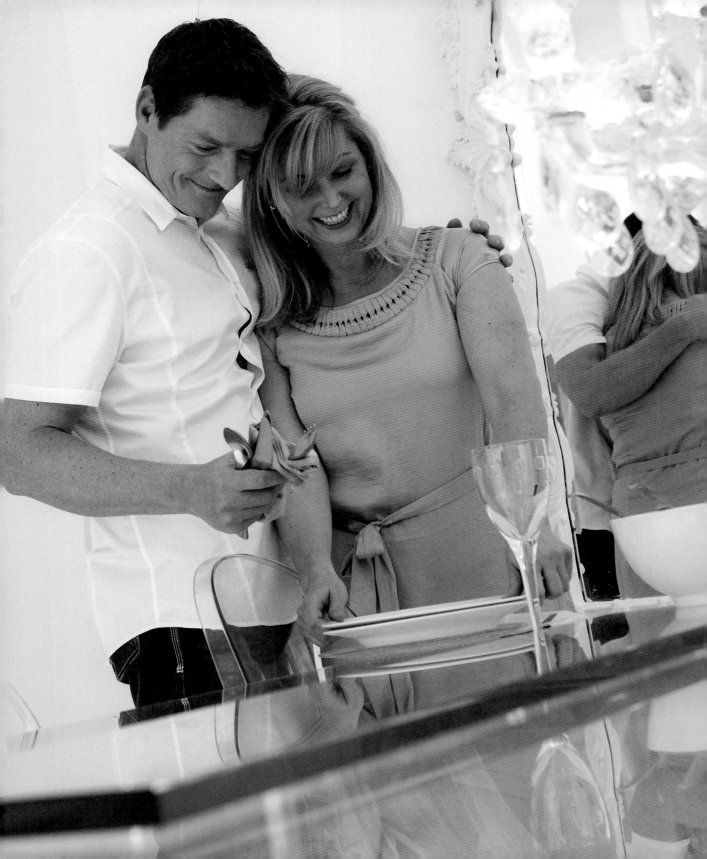

How much do you take responsibility for what happens in your life? For most of us, blaming others is more common than we realize. This is especially true when it comes to sex and romance. It is easy to point the finger at the opposite sex, yet this can be dangerous. In fact, it can prevent you from living the romantic life you want.

Yes, that's right—you can create romance. But first, you need to see what attitudes are holding you back. To start, answer the questions below and figure out just how often you play the blame game.

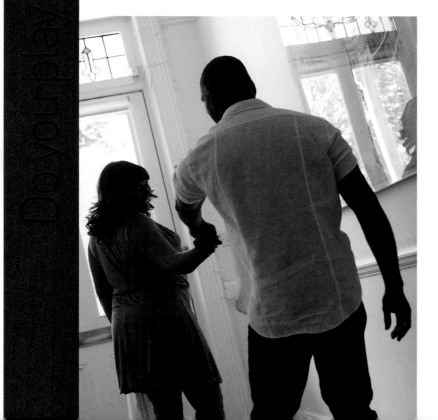

1 YOU GET TOGETHER WITH YOUR FRIENDS FOR A GIRLS' NIGHT OUT.

As usual, you sip cocktails and spend the night talking about:

Ⓐ Your ex from two years ago.

Ⓑ The dating service you recently joined and how awful it is.

Ⓒ The funny movie you just saw, your yoga class, your newest project at work, the ski trip you are planning for next winter, and your dating life.

2 THE HOLIDAYS ARE HERE!

Although you love turkey and all the trimmings, you dread the inevitable questions from your relatives about your continued singlehood. Thus, when Uncle Mac asked you for the third time, "Why are you still single?" you:

Ⓐ Jokingly reply "There's no one left—all the good ones are taken!"

Ⓑ Burst into tears and run from the room without saying a word.

Ⓒ Calmly state, "I appreciate your concern, but I actually prefer to keep my love life private," then gracefully change the subject.

3 YOUR PARTNER HASN'T MADE ANY SPECIAL PLANS

for date night, even though you have been hinting that you really want to try something new and romantic. You:

Ⓐ Play up your small headache and cancel your date night. You have laundry to catch up on anyway.

Ⓑ Pout silently throughout the dinner and movie, and say, "I'm fine" when he asks if you are okay.

C Make a reservation at a new restaurant on the other side of town and break out a sexy dress. If he doesn't know how to plan a great date, he can learn by example.

4 **YOUR KIDS ARE HYPER AND THE HOUSE IS A MESS.**
Your partner comes home from work, takes in all the chaos, and asks how he can help. You:
A Say "Everything is great! Go ahead and watch the game with your friends. I can handle this."
B Roll your eyes and snap, "Just make yourself useful, if possible. I don't have time to explain to you what to do to make life easier."
C Ask him to take the kids off your hands while you tidy up the kitchen. Then, when he comes home, he can empty the dishwasher while you play with the kids.

5 **YOU HAVE BEEN DATING A NEW GUY FOR THE LAST MONTH AND IT'S GOING GREAT.**
You are ready to take it to the next level. However, as you start getting intimate, he skips foreplay and heads right to the main event, leaving you unsatisfied and unhappy. You:
A Pretend to have an orgasm. He might not be great in bed, but it's hard meeting someone nice!

B Stop taking his calls immediately. You might have a lot in common, but you need a man, not a boy.
C Ask him if you can slow it down and show him what types of positions you like. Hey, someone has to teach him!

6 **YOU AND YOUR FAMILY LEAVE FOR A LONG WEEKEND AWAY.**
When you arrive at your resort, you:
A Smile as your partner settles in to catch up on Sportscenter while you slather sunscreen on the kids, round up the water toys, and head down to the pool to check out the slide.
B Grumble loudly about the lack of sunshine and the tiny bathroom.
C Organize a walk on the beach— your kids can collect the shells while you and your partner enjoy the sunset.

7 **YOU LEARN ON FRIDAY ABOUT A PRESENTATION FOR MONDAY MORNING.**
When your boss asks you to take the lead, you:
A Say, "Absolutely! I have plenty of time to pull this together."
B Agree to do it, then call your partner to complain about how you'll be at the office all weekend.
C Express your enthusiasm, but ask if you can take the following Friday morning off as comp time.

A-type answers mean that you frequently slip into blaming behavior, although you may not realize it. It may be difficult for you to express your needs, causing you to behave as if everything is fine even when you are upset. You might find yourself constantly striving to meet the needs of the people around you, while remaining unfulfilled and lonely. Verbalizing your needs will help you minimize blame.

B-type answers indicate that you may be stuck in the blame game, and often project your blame outward. Other people may perceive you as being sarcastic, or even bitter. This can prevent you from forming meaningful relationships and from creating the life you want.

C-type answers mean that you are in a healthier place. You work to keep your relationships happy and strong, and you aren't afraid to take the reins of your love life and direct it where you want it to go. Equally, you protect your quality of life and are open when you feel there needs to be a change.

❝ It is easy to point the finger at the opposite sex, but this can prevent you from living the life you want. **❞**

Reversing the blame game

It's Saturday night. You've had a big fight earlier in the day with your partner. In need of solace and understanding, you meet your girlfriends for martinis and spend the whole night talking about how "There are no good men out there," "Men just don't know how to treat a woman anymore," and "At our age, all the worthwhile men are taken."

Taking responsibility

Does the above story sound familiar? While there is nothing wrong with commiserating with your girlfriends about the struggles of matrimony or meeting Mr. Right, it can lead to a very harmful behavior—the blame game. We can all easily fall into this trap, believing that men have failed women, men can't meet our expectations, men don't understand us, and on and on and on. In some cases, these blanket accusations against the opposite sex might be true. But there is more than enough blame to go around, and if you don't examine the role you might be playing in your own unhappiness, you can never treat the real cause for it.

Instead of falling into this damaging cycle, try this: After an argument or a bad dating experience, spend some time reflecting on what you did to contribute to the miscommunication and the disagreement. It takes two to tango when it comes to a great relationship and the same is true for a bad one. That doesn't mean that you should become a martyr and blame yourself for everything that goes wrong, including the unpaid bills or the torrential downpour outside. But you can examine how your own behavior might have contributed to your unhappiness, and think about what changes might help protect your happiness in the future.

Although it might sound difficult—or even depressing—to look at your contribution to what's not working in your life, it can actually be quite empowering. When you take responsibility for your own behavior, you stop taking a passive role in your life, and instead gain control of your destiny. This means that your future is in your hands, instead of in the hands of the men you date, or in the hands of your boss or friends or family. It also means that positive change is truly possible. Once you stop blaming, you acknowledge that *you* are in charge—and that feels pretty good.

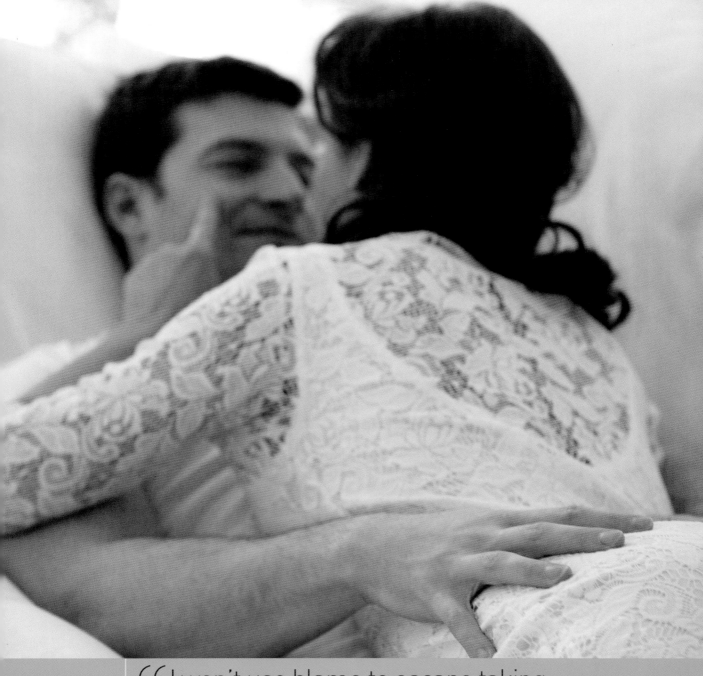

❝I won't use blame to escape taking control of my life or my relationships.❞

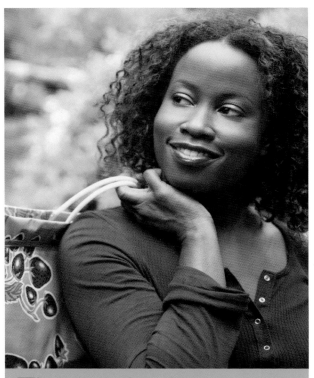

The truth about...

GETTING RID OF BLAME

When you are unhappy, it is easy to slip into blaming behavior, accusing your partner of not being understanding or romantic enough, or yourself of not being sexy or skinny enough. Taking action and making changes in your life isn't easy. It takes guts and determination. It's much easier (and safer) to sit around blaming other people for your problems.

However, when you drop the blame game and take the initiative to make your life better, you always succeed. Even if you don't accomplish your original goal, you succeed simply by being motivated and involved and open to all possibilities. You become the heroine of your life, rather than a mopey bystander.

Positivity and love

While a positive and proactive attitude is important in every relationship, it is especially key when it comes to finding and keeping love. Many women enter into the dating world on the defensive, either as a result of past relationships that have gone awry or as a natural by-product of the society in which we live. This is normal, but it can pose a huge obstacle to your happiness.

Perhaps you were hurt or abandoned in your own childhood by a key figure in your life. Maybe your last lover broke your heart in countless places. Even if you have been relatively unscathed in your life relationships, the media gives us a head start in the blame game, or at least lowers our expectations. From movies to television shows to women's magazines, we are inundated with messages that men are jerks. They forget your birthday, they cheat, they can't remember to take out the trash, and all they want to do is drink beer and watch football with their buddies. Popular culture trains you to look for these flaws in your own partner, and when you find them, your worst fears are validated.

The truth is this: If you expect to be let down by the ones you love, you always will be—and your relationship will take a major blow as a result. No relationship can thrive in an atmosphere of negativity. If you enter a relationship with the belief that men don't have the emotional intelligence or capability to treat you well, then you are setting yourself up for failure. An attitude that says, "I know you are going to hurt me, so I will shut you down before you get started" is not helpful for either of you. In fact, it almost guarantees that your communication will flounder and your partner won't be able to give you what you need.

Not only can a blaming attitude prevent you from connecting with your partner, it can also keep you from finding a date at all. Whether you are filling out an online dating form or walking your dog, people can read your attitude very quickly. If you seem like someone who is angry or insecure or not open to finding love, you will be met with the same negativity and reservations in others.

I'm not trying to judge you for the blame game. We all do it and we've all been taught to do it. I'm just asking you to look at where and when you are blaming others and consider an alternative response. This will help you see that the lens through which you view your relationship affects your behavior and your partner's behavior.

Identifying blaming behavior

As you read this, you might think, "That's not me. I don't blame others or look for flaws in my partner." However, blaming behavior can be very subversive. You often don't see it coming until it is too late. Some common ways that women blame men include:

The accusation: "I can't believe he has the nerve to check out the waitress in front of me!"
The truth: You are feeling insecure about your own appearance. Instead of admitting this, you make the easy, possibly incorrect, judgment that he is looking at other women. Remind yourself that your date chose to be at the restaurant with you, so there is no need to compare yourself to anyone else.

The accusation: "Doesn't he know tonight was supposed to be special? Why did he take me to the same restaurant we go to with the kids?"
The truth: In reality, it might not be that he wasn't feeling the romance, but that he didn't know what your expectation of romance was. You might think that having to spell out your needs for him isn't romantic, but spending the whole night pouting because he didn't meet your expectations isn't very romantic either. Teach him by example by taking charge of date-night plans yourself next time.

The accusation: "Our sex life is so boring. He never makes me feel sexy or tries anything new."

The truth: You have the power to change your sex life. If you want sex to be more passionate, you can be the catalyst for those changes (see page 140 for more on taking the reins of your sex life).

The accusation: "My sister's partner is so attentive, yet my boyfriend won't even ask about my day!"
The truth: You don't know everything that goes on in your sister's relationship, and it's not fair to judge your partner against someone else. Judgments like these cause you to view your relationship through a harmful and negative lens. Instead, be honest with your partner about your needs.

The accusation: "He has barely asked me a single question about myself all night. It's clear he is self-centered just like my last boyfriend."
The truth: Maybe you gravitate toward the talkative type. Or maybe your partner is distracted because he had a stressful day. If you assume rather than ask, you'll never know. And if you want his attention, enter the conversation with confidence and share about your life without being asked.

By identifying and removing this type of blame from your relationship, you will find it easier to appreciate your partner—or at least easier to give him the benefit of the doubt. This is the first step toward becoming empowered to move forward in a happier, healthier relationship.

> **❝** Blaming behavior can be very subversive. You often don't see it coming until it is too late. **❞**

Examining self-blame

There is a flip side to blaming behavior that can be just as harmful as blaming others—blaming yourself, known as "self-blame." It's important to examine the things that you consistently feel guilty about, then work to banish these concerns from your thought cycle as much as possible.

Gaining perspective

We spend hours, days, even years brooding over our perceived failings and mistakes. Every woman has something that triggers self-blame. Perhaps you feel guilty that you spend so much time at work instead of with the kids, or you feel ashamed that you no longer fit into a size two, or you worry that you don't initiate sex as often as you used to.

Generally, we experience feelings of guilt because we think we "should" have done something differently or we "should" behave, look, or think in a different way. Whether you're measuring yourself against a Hollywood celebrity, a neighbor, or even a younger version of yourself, these comparisons can be devastating for you and your relationship.

And, perhaps not surprisingly, women may be programmed to feel more guilt and regret than men. In a recent study, researchers questioned almost 300 men and women about the situations that left them feeling guilty, from small things such as forgetting to send a birthday card to larger, life-changing things, like cheating on one's partner.

The results showed that women worried far more about hurting other people, while men seemed to feel guilt most often when it came to their own needs, such as eating or drinking too much. In most situations, women were more likely to brood over their behavior and be angry with themselves.

Rethinking your "should" list

Identifying the thoughts that make you feel guilty helps you rid your life of self-blame. Consider some common "shoulds" that haunt women everyday:

● **I feel so guilty** giving the kids lunch money again today. I should make them a homemade lunch like the other moms in the neighborhood.

● **I can't believe** I have only lost 2 pounds after I've been dieting for a month. I should be so much thinner by now.

● **I should have worn** something dressier for our date. Now I feel so dowdy compared to all the other women in the restaurant.

Overcoming self-blame

All of these "shoulds" slowly chip away at our happiness and self-esteem. If you are undergoing a constant mental beating, you won't feel empowered to make the changes you want in your life, and you won't be able to live in the moment or enjoy time with your partner. Instead, you will be thinking of all the things you "should" be doing. Imagine how this affects not only your relationship, but also your sex life. Having sex with a to-do list in your head, along with a side of guilt? Not exactly orgasm material!

The lesson? Take a cue from your partner and make it a point not to worry about the little things. Maybe your house isn't perfectly clean, or you didn't have a chance to cook a gourmet meal for your weekend dinner party. Take the focus off those small details by appreciating the bigger picture— such as that your house really feels like a home, or your potluck plans allowed friends to share recipes. Studies show that people who practice gratitude on a daily basis are more likely to have a positive attitude, which means that you will be more likely to receive positive attention from those around you.

When you are at peace with who you are, you are much more likely to attract appreciation and respect, whether it's with a long-term partner or a new love interest. This can only happen when you end a pattern of self-blame. You must make the decision every day to accept yourself and the world around you, and to leave blame, regret, and guilt at the door. Every day you make that decision, you will be rewarded with healthy, happy relationships.

The other side of should

Denying yourself small pleasures to avoid feelings of guilt can be just as damaging as dwelling on the things you think you should have accomplished. Reflect on this list of things women often give up due to feelings of guilt—then do your best to banish all such self-accusatory thoughts.

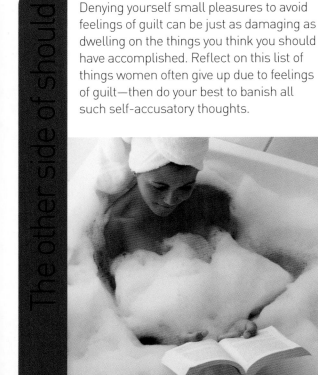

I shouldn't

● **Order dessert.** Self-blame thought: "I am already overweight. I don't deserve dessert."
● **Speak my mind.** "I will sound stupid."
● **Make the first move in the bedroom.** "Nice girls don't do that. I will seem too forward."
● **Leave the kids at home.** "It's more important that the kids are happy than that we go out on a date."
● **Spend free time with my friends.** "I should devote my time and energy to our relationship."
● **Have a hot bath.** "Taking care of the house is more important than having time to myself every day."
● **Spend money on myself.** "I won't be a good mom if I don't put our kids first."
● **Tell him what I need in the bedroom.** "Talking openly about my sexual needs isn't feminine."

Shifting your perspective

A lucky truth is that your thoughts and your emotions are really under your control. Once you realize this, they won't have such negative power over you. While you can't control the weather, the traffic, or the people around you, you can control how you react to these things, and refuse to get caught in a cycle of blame. And that means you can decide to turn a bad day into a good day any time you choose.

Choosing positivity

Unfortunately, it isn't always easy to recognize when we are caught in blaming behavior, either toward our partner or ourselves. For most of us, the blame game is ingrained, something we learned from our parents or our peers. In fact, most people blame, blame, blame all day long: "My boss was in one of his moods," or "Traffic was awful; it took me an hour to get home," or "I was in a perfectly fine mood until my partner was late for our dinner date."

In each of the above statements, the speaker is diminishing her own power by attributing her bad mood to factors outside of her control. It would be rare indeed to be in a good mood if the rest of the world had a say in it! There will always be days that include grumpy bosses, bad traffic, and delayed dates, but that doesn't have to translate into a negative—or blaming—state of mind.

Although it seems like all of the occurrences above are out of your control, the truth is that at any point during the day, you can decide to shift. You can actually decide to have a good day, partners and coworkers and traffic regardless. All you have to do is *shift*.

Making the shift

The best way to improve your attitude is to recognize that you need a new perspective, and then do something about it. Try these tips to start:

Notice that you are stuck in a bad mood. Start by simply becoming aware that you feel powerless over your mood. While it can help to know why you feel upset, ultimately the reason doesn't really matter. The real problem is that you are interpreting the world around you in a way that creates anger. Recognizing that you are in a bad mood is often enough to help you begin to move on. Don't judge yourself or become upset with yourself. Bad moods strike everyone, and it's nothing to feel guilty about.

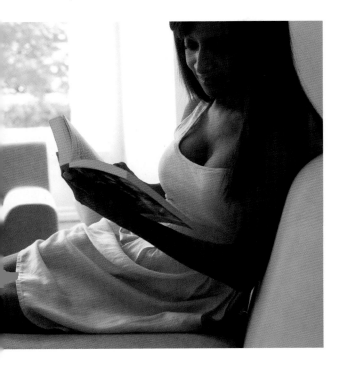

Personalize your treatment. Make a list of ways to release negative feelings. Maybe it's listening to music, or exercising. Find out what calms you down and make it a priority to work it into your day.

Overcoming worry

You can kill irrational worries with a similar step-by-step approach. When you are stuck in a negative thought pattern, the first step is to figure out what thoughts are creating the sadness or fear or anger. Recognize that you are stuck, then consider these four questions from Byron Katie's self-help program, "The Work," to help you make a positive shift (for more on "The Work," see Bibliography, page 248).

- Is it true?
- Can you absolutely know that it's true?
- How do you react—what happens—when you believe that thought?
- Who would you be without the thought?

Figure out what is going on inside your head.
Take a step back from the situation. Are you upset because you think your coworker takes advantage of you? Do you feel like everyone around you is incompetent? Once you figure out your thought pattern, you can decide if it has merit.

Pay attention to your body language. If you're feeling angry you'll probably notice that your arms are on your hips, or that they're crossed. If you are sad, you may be hunched over. Moving your body out of its current position will actually help shift your perspective and your mood. In fact, experts in this area recommend what they call "creative joint play." It seems silly, but it helps you shift. Here's how to do it: stand up, and move every joint in your body in all different directions. You may feel crazy at first, but it really works.

Asking yourself these questions can help put your thoughts into context. For example, if you are angry that your partner didn't help clean the house, you may be thinking, "My partner doesn't care about my needs or how busy I am." In this moment, ask yourself: Is it true that he doesn't care about my needs? Is it absolutely true? Or, is it more likely that he simply didn't know you were planning to clean? See if you can find an explanation that seems more realistic then your initial, emotion-based thought.

Look at the feelings that stem from your reaction: you feel angry and hurt. Yet how would you feel if it wasn't true? If the problem is not that your partner doesn't care about you, what would your behavior be like? Would you be able to overlook a minor household issue and simply try to be clear about your needs next time? By reacting rationally instead of emotionally, you are more likely to put a smaller issue into context—and stop the blame game before it gets out of control.

Living in the present

Even after you have practiced shifting perspective, little things about your partner can still cause conflict—the way he slurps his soup, the way he cracks his knuckles, his annoying habit of being late for everything. Again, this is blaming behavior rearing its ugly head. There is a reason why you didn't notice these annoying qualities when you were first dating. It's sad but true: as a relationship progresses, you naturally have less patience and gratitude for your partner.

You spot it, you got it

Interestingly enough, the things we nitpick in our partners are often the things we don't like in ourselves. This is the theory of "you spot it, you got it." In other words, our own flaws are always the easiest to see in someone else. For example, if you are unhappy with your own weight, you might find yourself making sarcastic comments when your partner reaches for a third helping of pizza. If you are feeling stressed about the kids, you might suddenly start complaining about your partner's parenting skills. It all comes down to one thing: You don't like the lack of control you have over your own life, so you focus on the lack of control your partner seems to have over his life. Subconsciously, it always seems easier to try to get your partner to change than to try to change yourself.

Unfortunately, even if your partner were to become the perfect husband, parent, lover, employee, gym buff, or whatever else you believe you need from him, it still wouldn't give you back that sense of control. Your partner's perfection can only go so far—you are the only one who can ultimately make yourself happy.

Becoming what you need

The next time you catch yourself ready to make a sarcastic comment about your partner's bad table manners or lack of fashion sense, stop and ask yourself what it is within that is trying to find its way out. You will likely find that it is not just your partner's soup-slurping. Maybe what you are really feeling is that your partner has become complacent, or that your time together doesn't feel romantic—and that, by extension, you don't feel special.

The best way to turn that voice off and get what you need is to become what you need. Shooting off a nasty comment to your partner won't make either of you happy, nor is it likely to change anything about your relationship. Thinking about how you can inspire more romance in your relationship can create change, however.

To do this, first think about what would be romantic for you. Then, consider what would feel pleasurable for your partner. If you're like most couples, atmosphere and emotional connection will be very important for you, while direct visual stimulation will be very important for him. The good news? When you're planning the romance, you can incorporate both. For example, try drawing a bath, lighting some candles, and inviting your partner to get naked with you. Regularly planning moments like these will get both of your hearts racing—and can help put an end to petty disagreements.

The quick fix

In the meantime, though, what are you supposed to do about that soup-slurping? Take a deep breath and get back in the moment. Let go of the bad day that is still haunting you. Remind yourself why you love your partner. Don't stick to general things like "He is smart" or "He is nice." Think specifically, such as "I love how he makes funny faces" or "I love that he calls me by pet names."

If you still can't shake it (after all, some days it's very hard to be in the present), get up and leave the room for a few minutes. When you come back, the soup course will be over, and you will have saved yourself an unnecessary argument (see page 226 for more ideas on how to shift your thought process).

Also, remember: you spot it, you got it. The next time you become irritated at your partner's behavior, examine yourself. (Hint: The more forcefully you think "No way am I guilty of that!" the more likely it is that your behaviors are similar.) If you seek to understand and compare your behavior patterns, you'll gain a greater sense of empathy for each other and become a little less sensitive.

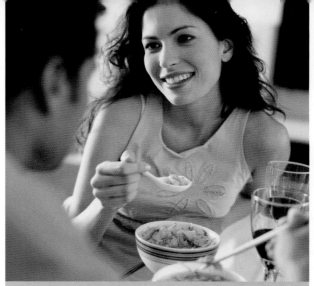

How to...

INJECT SPONTANEITY INTO YOUR LOVE LIFE

You can also reverse the "you spot it, you got it" theory. If there is a trait you wish you saw in your partner's life, consider how you could exhibit that trait yourself. For example, if you are craving more romance and spontaneity, be purposeful about creating some. Here's one way to do this.

1 Book a hotel room on an ordinary Tuesday night without telling your partner.

2 Tell him you have dinner reservations, and, over the wine and appetizers, let him know that you have booked a romantic hotel room for the night.

3 Enjoy the knowledge that you have made his week—and also increased the chances of him surprising you in the near future. Once he sees how sexy and spontaneous you can be, he will be much more likely to act spontaneously himself.

4 Bonus: When you see how appreciative he is, you will start to see yourself as he does—as an irresistible woman who can easily inspire romance.

Rethinking Mr. Right

If you are single, you have likely thought up a few must-have qualities for your future partner. For instance, your list might include a partner who is at least six feet tall, makes a certain amount of money each year, or has a full head of hair. Be careful as you write your list. No matter how innocent these must-haves may seem, they have the potential to stand in the way of you and love.

Evaluating your list

As you read this and mentally cling to your list, ask yourself why you are set on certain qualities. Why does your partner need to have a certain profession? (Is it possible that what you really want, rather than a lawyer or a doctor, is a smart, ambitious partner?) Why does he have to be a head taller than you? (Is it because you "should" be shorter and therefore more feminine than your partner?)

If you sit down and really think about why you are hanging on to certain specifications, you might be surprised to find that they don't have a very firm foundation. While some things on your list may be sound, there are often many more that are superficial and won't really impact your happiness in a relationship. In fact, even some of the criteria

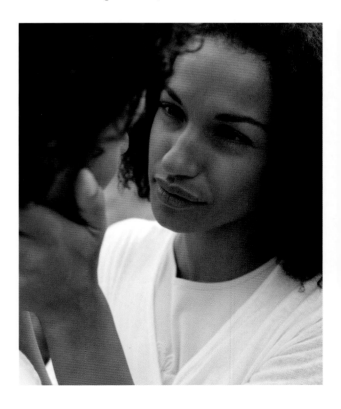

that seem sound might not hold water when you really think about them. For instance, if you have decided that you don't want your partner to have kids from another relationship, think about why. Is it that you don't like the idea of him having other financial commitments? Do you think that kids will take time away from you? Consider whether these reasons are really deal-breakers for you.

Also, spend some time thinking objectively about the positive side of the situation. Perhaps having kids has taught him important lessons about responsibility and consistency, and given him a glimpse of what unconditional love can look like. Try to look at the whole picture before you let any one reason rule a potential partner out.

The bottom line is that your list for Mr. Right can become another excuse to play the blame game. If you tend to get hung up on the "negative" qualities of every single guy you meet, you are essentially blaming each of these men for not being the real-life incarnation of your idealized list. If you want to find the right relationship, you have to be willing to accept someone, flaws and all.

Creating the "real" list

By uncovering the true motivation behind your list, you can strike out unnecessary stipulations that are holding you back from finding true love. Your list should really only include a handful of "must-haves," such as that your partner loves you and respects you. Remember that you have friends with different backgrounds, personalities, and beliefs—so why would you assume that your perfect match will be someone that you can predict and control?

The next time you catch yourself dismissing someone because he is too short, thin, outspoken, or different from you, stop and give him another chance. Mr. Right comes in very unlikely packages—you just have to take the time to unwrap him.

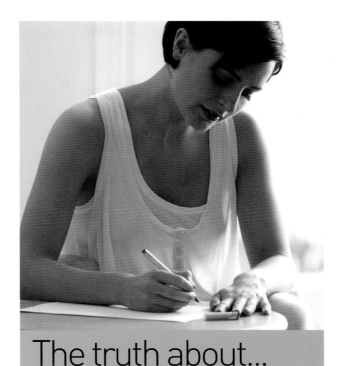

The truth about...

YOUR MR. RIGHT

In order to create a list of qualities that are really important to you, think about what draws you to your best friends. These same qualities are likely the ones that you should seek in a life partner. For example, does your best friend have a great sense of humor? Is she open-minded and passionate? This is an easy way for you to separate real qualities from superficial qualities like "He has a six-pack!"

Prioritizing the items on your list is also useful. Arrange your list in order of importance. For instance, is intelligence more important than height? Then, cross out everything beyond number five on the list of your priorities. They are probably requirements that you can live without.

Understanding relationship roles

When you are playing the blame game, you often get stuck in certain roles. Especially during conflict, it is tempting to react from a mental script, without truly thinking through your actions and words. When this happens, you get stuck blaming your partner or yourself for the conflict, instead of examining the root causes of the argument or expressing your authentic needs. Learning to identify the roles you choose is a good way to stop the blame game in action.

Identifying your roles

It's easy to get stuck in a certain role, especially if you have been in a relationship for a long time. Just as you discover certain ways of managing chores and errands, you also discover ways of managing emotions. This is true for every couple, and it is harmful if it means that these emotions are not fully dealt with and thus never get resolved.

When you are stuck in negative roles, you won't be able to express your needs to your partner honestly, and you won't be open to hearing his needs. Authentic communication can only occur when you both agree to get out of your comfort zones and express your true needs. This isn't always easy, but you will be shocked when you discover how quickly you can resolve arguments once you stop being trapped by tradition.

The victim role

Everyone slips into the victim role from time to time. Whenever you take a passive role in your life and your relationship, and experience your actions as the effect of someone or something else, you are playing the victim. This impacts the way you interact with your partner, and the way he thinks about you. Common victim behavior includes:

Taking a passive role in situations, yet being upset by the outcome. Example: Saying you don't know where you want to go for dinner, but becoming angry when your partner chooses a place you don't like.

Being sensitive or easily injured; always requiring apologies; looking for hidden insults; needing to be comforted before your good mood can be restored. Example: When your partner asks you if you plan on going to the gym the next day, you take it to mean he thinks you are overweight—when he really just wants to know your schedule for the upcoming day.

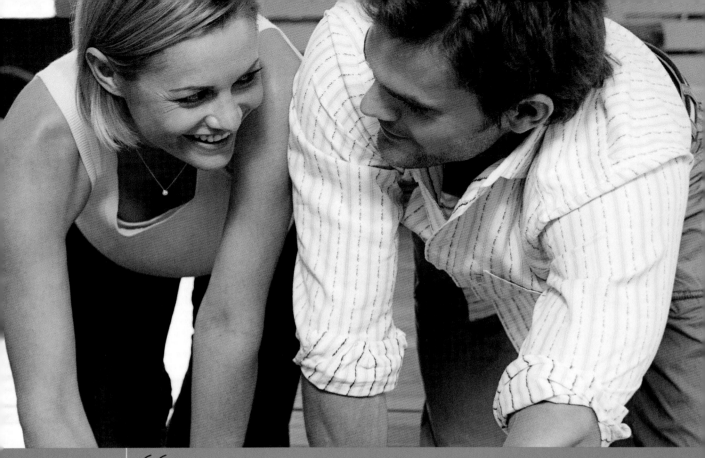

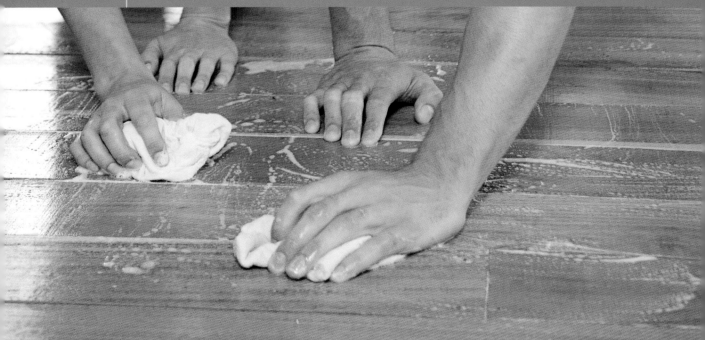

PERSONAL
AFFIRMATION

❝I will ask my partner for help when I need it, and tell him when I am upset.❞

> **❝**Once you begin to notice specific behaviors that you fall back on, you can let go of the role.**❞**

Frequently saying "I can't" or "I need your help." While it is good to be able to express your needs and ask for help, victims sometimes use this as a way to avoid taking responsibility for their lives. Example: Saying you can't communicate with your partner, and giving up without trying.

Once you begin to notice specific victim behaviors that you fall back on, you can let go of the role, and adopt a more authentic mode of communication (for more on abandoning old roles, see box at right).

The villain role

The villain is critical, sarcastic, and always has to be right. When you are in the villain role, you are often hiding insecurity. Rather than showing this vulnerability and communicating honestly about your hurt or your fear, you feign confidence and try to attack your partner. Your partner might accommodate your role, and he might even be intimidated by your show of power, but every time you adopt the villain role, you drive a wedge into your relationship and weaken your bond. Read on for common villain behavior, then check out the box at right to see how to move beyond it.

Attacking your partner for things out of his control.
Example: Traffic is backed up and you are going to be late for dinner. You say: "I told you we should have left earlier, but you never listen to me!"

Criticizing his character rather than his behavior.
Example: He didn't get you a Valentine's Day gift, and you accuse him of not caring about you.

Trying to make your partner feel inferior.
Example: He doesn't understand why you are upset about something, and rather than explain, you act exasperated, saying that he never understands you unless you spell out your thought process.

Refusing to admit wrongdoing or drop an argument.
Example: The argument is over and you are making up, but still you feel compelled to say, "I just hope I made my point really clear. You really upset me today. I am still kind of in shock about it."

The hero role

When you are in the hero role, you go out of your way to make sure everyone around you is happy no matter the cost to you. This is a very common role for women, who often naturally feel that it is their job to make sure that everyone in the household has every need met. Remember, though, that your needs are just as important.

From the outside, when you are in the hero role, you look like the ideal wife and mother. On the inside, however, you are stressed, exhausted, and completely separated from your inner sensuality and joy. Moreover, when you take on all the responsibility in the household, you infantilize your partner, instead of treating him like your equal in all things. This will negatively affect your relationship and your attraction to each other. On your end, you will likely become frustrated with how little he steps up. You may even stop desiring sex with him because he no longer seems like a "man." On his end, he will begin to feel resentment toward you, and will shut down, feeling like he can do no right. Often he will also lose his libido, as a result of feeling emasculated and disconnected. Some of the most common hero behaviors include:

Taking on way more than you can handle and refusing to ask for help. Example: You work a 10-hour day, then come home and sweep the kitchen, make the kids their lunches, and fold the laundry. When your husband asks if you need any help, you say "No, thanks. I got it!"

Allowing your partner to forgo responsibility in the relationship. Example: When your partner won't communicate with you or open up, you blame it on yourself, saying, "I shouldn't have pushed him so hard. I can communicate enough for the both of us!"

Treating your partner like he is incompetent. Example: You have to go out of town to visit family for a few days. Instead of trusting him to take care of the house and the kids, you leave a million lists and reminders, and call every hour to check in.

The bottom line is that you need to work as a team in order for your relationship to thrive. Slow down, ask for help, and stop trying to do it all. When you are aware of yourself slipping into a hero role, acknowledge it and move on by saying something such as, "You know, honey? I could use some help in the kitchen. And, after dinner, let's swap turns watching the kids."

Roles and blaming

All of these roles can contribute to the blame game, because they prevent you from communicating honestly. This means blame can creep in and take over. As a victim and a villain you tend to blame everyone around you, and, as a hero, you tend to take all the blame on yourself.

To avoid this version of the blame game, try to stay aware of when you slip into a role, and ask your partner to let you know when he sees you taking on these old habits. This checks-and-balances system will keep you both on track and moving forward, out of damaging communication patterns.

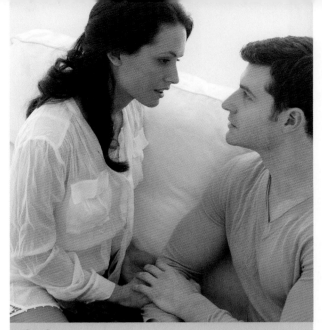

How to...

ABANDON OLD ROLES

The truth is that it's not possible to totally remove damaging roles from your relationship, as these patterns have been ingrained into our personalities over the years. What you can do is learn how to work through them in a way that brings healing and resolution. Here's how:

1 When you feel yourself getting upset, take a few minutes to yourself. Breathe deeply.

2 Try to identify your primary emotions and the stories behind them. Are you scared because your partner snapped at you? Are you angry because he forgot your birthday, and you feel like he doesn't really care about you?

3 Sort out why you are truly upset, and then explain your reasons calmly and clearly. When you speak "unarguably," sharing your feelings and the stories behind them, it becomes much easier to shift out of any damaging roles (see page 178 for more on speaking unarguably).

The opposite of blame

The bottom-line law of relationships is that you get what you give. Your partner will almost always reflect your own attitude right back at you. As you rid your life of blame, you will make room for more effective and positive modes of communication, such as praise. Praise has the opposite effect of blame. A healthy dose of praise, or appreciation, in a relationship can make it virtually impossible for blame to thrive.

Learning to praise

Praise can have many different forms. A simple "You look great!" can go a long way, as can "Thanks for emptying the dishwasher," but praise can also be more multifaceted. Just remember to keep it genuine, personal, and frequent. Make it a goal to compliment or praise your partner at least twice a day. The more praise fills your relationship, the less room there will be for blame and bitterness. Here are some unique ways you can praise your partner:

Brag about him to your friends and your family. When you regularly look for the good qualities in your partner, it becomes easier to see them yourself. Tell your mother how he took care of you while you were sick, or share with a coworker how he watched the kids while you went out with your girlfriends. When you make gratitude a daily habit, it will noticeably change your attitude toward him.

Reaffirm his role in the family. Although it might not be readily obvious, men take a lot of pride in their role in the family. Biological and social cues have trained him to see himself as the protector of you and your brood. When you compliment his skills as a father or husband, you are reaffirming his identity and boosting his masculinity. Tell him, "I love watching you play with the kids. They are so lucky to have such an amazing dad," or, "You can always cheer me up when I have a bad day. I love being your wife," or, "I was so touched by the way you went over and cut your mom's grass today. You take such good care of her; your dad would be proud." Nothing boosts a man's ego like knowing that he is fulfilling his role in the family.

Ask him for advice. People love to be needed, especially by their partners. If you show your partner that you need him (and not just for traditionally "male" tasks like taking out the trash and killing spiders), he will feel more secure and happy in your relationship. Do so by asking his advice about your worries, whether it is a fight you had with your best friend, a concern with the kids, or a managerial issue you are having at work. Knowing that you respect his opinion enough to seek it out can revolutionize the relationship for him.

Tell him that you want him. If you want to pay the ultimate compliment to a man, tell him that you want him—now, if possible! Knowing that you are attracted to him and fantasizing about being with him in the bedroom is the biggest ego boost for a man. Send him a text early in the day that simply says: "I can't stop thinking about you." Follow up later that afternoon with a more detailed email or phone call that outlines all the sexy details that you have on your mind.

Show him that you want him. Write an erotic short story starring you and your partner (or thinly veiled versions of you two). Leave it on his pillow, or in his briefcase. Include all your fantasies and the things you want to do with him. Later that night, take the iniative to make your fantasies a reality. This is one gift he won't soon forget!

Enjoy the time you spend with him. When someone loves your company, it boosts your self-esteem. Every good relationship is based on a good friendship. Let your partner know that you enjoy the time you spend together by setting your date night in stone and turning off your phone to give him your full attention. Enjoying his company, laughing at his jokes, and simply taking pleasure in your partnership is perhaps the best affirmation there is for him and for your relationship. As long as you can have fun together, you can survive almost anything.

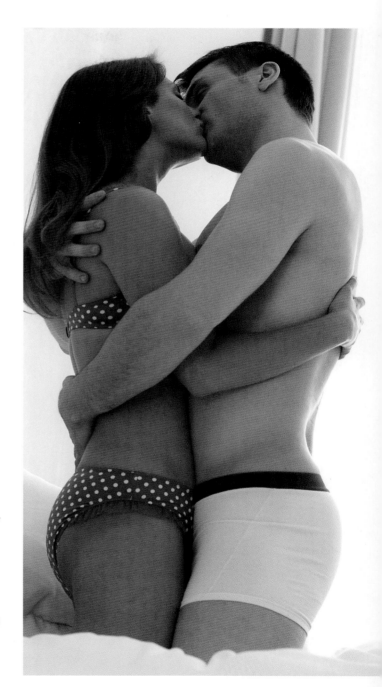

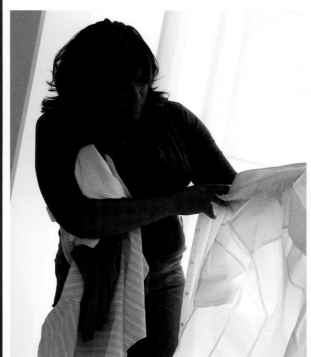 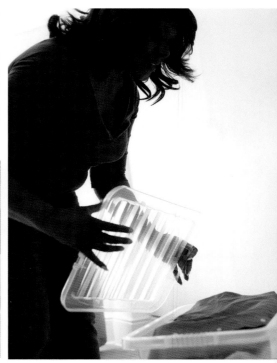

Chapter 2

Breaking the pattern

Relationship habits are hard to break. This isn't always a bad thing—in fact, understanding your own unique habits can provide valuable clues as to what you need in a relationship, and why. The factors that influence your pattern of attraction come from childhood, from your early relationships, and from the model set by your parents and other influential adults. Unraveling your past will help you move forward to a healthy relationship future.

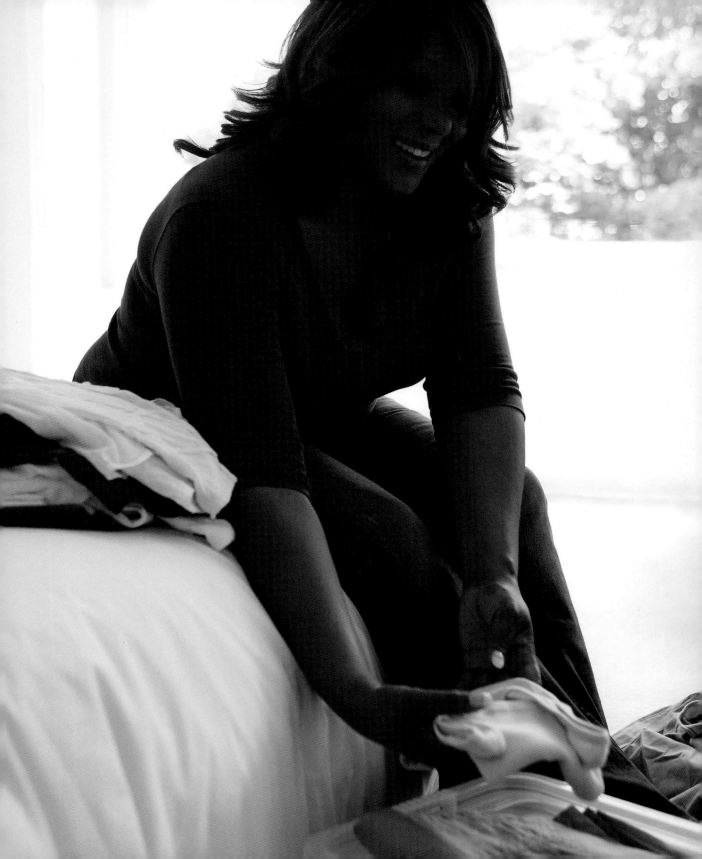

Do you follow a relationship pattern? If you're like most of us, the answer is yes. Our relationship histories—romantic, familial, even workplace relationships—have a huge impact on the status and satisfaction of our love lives. This is because all of these relationships reflect our core beliefs about what true love and companionship look like.

To examine where you stand, respond honestly to this questionnaire, acknowledging any questions that make you feel tense or uncomfortable.

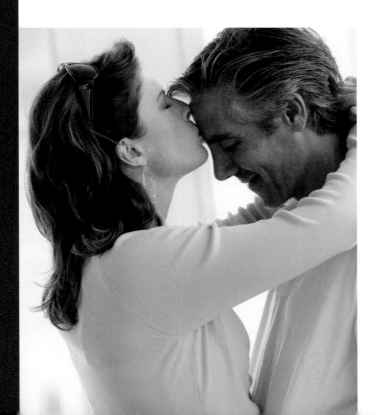

1 A CLOSE FRIEND WANTS TO SET YOU UP WITH HER COWORKER.

She shows you a picture and tells you how amazing he is—kind, smart, funny, and available. You:

A Shrug it off, and keep giving your friend excuses. He doesn't meet all your requirements. You need Mr. Right, not a poor substitute.

B Tell her to send him your number. You are always open to meeting cute, available guys!

C Tell her you will think about it, but internally dismiss him. You need a bad boy, not a boring corporate guy.

2 YOU AND YOUR SISTER ARE GOING SHOPPING FOR HER WEDDING DRESS.

While in the store, you:

A Show her the spreadsheet you made of different dresses and their cost. No sense in wasting time or money driving all over town.

B Help her look for dresses, and enjoy touching the fabrics and thinking about when your big day will come.

C Bring up the time she was overweight in junior high, and then get in a huge argument over the color of your bridesmaid dress.

3 IT'S FRIDAY NIGHT, AND YOU CAN'T WAIT TO COME HOME AND RELAX AFTER A GRUELING WEEK.

All you want to do is have a glass of wine and watch a movie with your partner. However, the house is a mess and your laundry has piled up. You:

Ⓐ Forgo your relaxation and clean the house top to bottom. It's too hard to relax in that chaos.
Ⓑ Decide to clean the house tomorrow morning. You desperately need a break, and the dirty socks are really not that pressing.
Ⓒ Shove everything in a nearby closet and forget about it.

4 YOUR PARENTS' MARRIAGE WAS NOT A HEALTHY ONE.

Even though they have been cordial to each other since the divorce, you still find yourself emotional and confused when you remember that painful, tense time. Years later, your own marriage is:
Ⓐ Painfully quiet. If your partner saw you angry or emotional he might not be able to take it and leave you.
Ⓑ Relatively peaceful. You have arguments, but nothing out of control.
Ⓒ Intense and passionate. From yelling to breaking dishes, your relationship is always rife with drama.

5 YOUR ADORABLE NIECE AND NEPHEW ARE COMING TO STAY WITH YOU FOR THE LONG WEEKEND.

When they arrive, you:
Ⓐ Immediately start picking up after them, and remind them to be careful on the new carpet.

Ⓑ Cover them with kisses and let them drag you outside to play tag in the backyard.
Ⓒ Let them watch TV past their bedtime and eat fast food, despite your sister's strict instructions.

6 YOU CAN HARDLY REMEMBER A TIME WHEN YOU HAVE BEEN SINGLE.

Looking back over your past relationships, you realize that:
Ⓐ You have basically dated the same guy since high school—outgoing and charming. All of these guys have made a great impression on your friends and family. The only problem is that they have a hard time making you a priority.
Ⓑ The men you've dated have been different in appearance and interests, but they were all intelligent and kind.
Ⓒ Your type is passionate, but also a bit rebellious and irresponsible.

7 WHAT ROLE DO YOU USUALLY PLAY IN A ROMANTIC RELATIONSHIP?

When you think about it, you realize:
Ⓐ You like to play the hero and solve every problem for your partner.
Ⓑ You truly try to be yourself and make choices that fit well with your long-term goals.
Ⓒ You crave romance, and walk away from any relationship that feels stale.

A-type answers may mean that you are stuck in controlling behavior. You want to perfect the world around you, and you want everything to be "just so." Unfortunately, this means that you miss out on a lot of fun and aren't open to meeting new people or having new experiences.

B-type answers indicate that, for the most part, you are in a healthy place and have found a good combination of working hard and playing hard. Life is probably more fun for you, and while you occasionally get stressed out, you can usually roll with the punches and enjoy life. This makes it a lot easier and more natural to find and grow good love.

C-type answers suggest that you are stuck in an unhealthy relationship routine. You probably haven't been able to move on from the past, and you tend to sweep things under the rug rather than face them head-on in a healthy way. If you are afraid to take the bull by the horns and seize life's opportunities for fun and love, it's going to be very hard to find and keep the relationship you want.

66 Our relationship histories have a huge impact on the status and satisfaction of our love lives. 99

Examining relationship patterns

Do you ever feel like you keep getting stuck in the same bad relationship over and over again? At first, everything starts out great. The passion is there, the sex is amazing, and you start to think he might be the one. But then, red flags begin to appear. He starts getting jealous and snooping through your things. He tries to control how much time you spend with friends, and he makes derogatory comments about your weight or fashion sense. On top of it all, you can't help but get the eerie feeling that you have been down this road before.

Defining repetition compulsion

Chances are, you have probably found yourself stuck in repetitive relationship patterns. This replaying is known as "repetition compulsion" in the therapy world. Repetition compulsion is a psychological phenomenon in which a person unconsciously relives or recreates a traumatic event or its circumstances over and over again. This includes reenacting the event or putting oneself in situations where there is a high probability of the event occurring again.

The concept of repetition compulsion was first coined by Sigmund Freud, who believed that there are two ways to relive your past: 1) through memories, or 2) through actions, the latter being the basis of repetition compulsion. There are many different ways this repetition compulsion can play out in a person's life. For instance, someone who was spanked as a child may incorporate spanking into his or her adult sexual practices. Or, a victim of childhood sexual abuse from an older friend or relative may attempt to seduce another person of authority in his or her life, such as a boss, therapist, or any other type of mentor.

Why would a person want to relive or reenact a painful memory? Most therapists believe that this unhealthy repetition could be an attempt to master and thus overcome one's negative experiences. Since a person cannot go back in time and undo hurtful memories, he or she subconsciously (or, at times, consciously) tries to repeat those experiences. In doing so, the person hopes to master the experience and gain a positive outcome, thus becoming victorious over the past. The ending, however, is unfortunately rarely a happy one, and the person usually ends up repeating the same destructive behaviors and relationships over and over again, without moving forward in the way he or she subconsciously hopes to do.

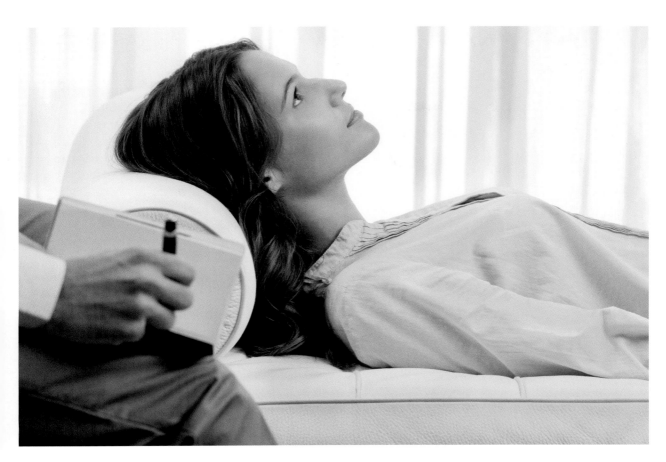

Real-life example: Nicole's story

Nicole's story is a good example of repetition compulsion. Like many people, Nicole's childhood was troubled and this greatly impacted her ability to form healthy relationships. Now, she is a 30-year-old receptionist living in Boston. After a brief marriage in her early 20s that ended due to physical abuse, Nicole has been looking for love. Her friends have tried to set her up with nice men, but she doesn't feel a spark with them: Her kind of guy is a bit rough around the edges. Her relationships are heated and passionate, but things always unravel and the man becomes controlling and abusive.

After her divorce, Nicole swore she would never allow herself to be hurt again, but she continually finds herself in relationships where she gets pushed around, both physically and emotionally. Her friends tell her that she ends up in these situations because she craves drama, but Nicole knows that isn't true. She doesn't want drama, she wants real, lasting love—and she doesn't know why she can't find it.

After some encouragement from her mother, Nicole agrees to see a therapist. While there, Nicole discusses her history. The therapist asks Nicole about her father, whom Nicole hasn't seen for 20 years. Nicole opens up about how her father was an alcoholic and abused her mother, but she is quick to point out that her father never laid a hand on her. Because she did not suffer any direct physical abuse, Nicole doesn't think her father's behavior could rightly have any effect on her. However, with her therapist's help, Nicole is able to understand that growing up in that environment greatly affected her. She spent her formative years learning that men should be loud and controlling. Though her father never laid a hand on her, he set her up for future abuse by causing her to subconsciously believe that abuse is a form of passion. No wonder Nicole never went for the nice guys she was introduced to—she didn't feel a spark because there was no potential for violence, which her history taught her was the definition of attraction.

Nicole was seeking out violent relationships because she associated abuse with love. She was also attempting to make peace with the past. Her repetitive-compulsive fantasy was that if she was lovable and understanding enough, then she would change the abuser or heal him, which she was unable to do as a child. Subconsciously, she felt that this would make her "good," something she was unable to believe as a child. Sadly, when it didn't work, she only ended up with more abuse and pain, which further harmed her self-esteem and trust.

By becoming aware of her reasons for choosing the wrong men, and through continued work with her therapist, Nicole was able to meet someone who was both passionate and kind. Though she still struggles with accepting her traumatic childhood, she is finally able to understand that she deserves to be in a relationship without violence.

Repetition compulsion doesn't only occur in romantic relationships. You might find yourself repeating patterns with toxic friends or family members, or getting stuck in an unhealthy cycle at work. All of these things will affect your relationship because they impact your self-esteem, your mood, and your general well-being. See right for a list of common repetitive-compulsive behaviors.

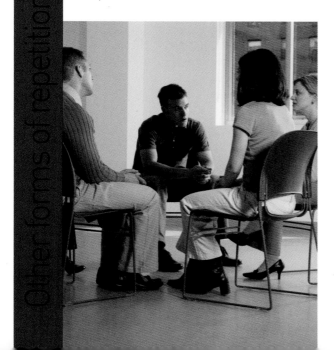

Patterns of addiction

- Alcoholism/drug abuse
- Emotional eating
- Anorexia/bulimia
- Exercise bulimia
- OCD rituals
- Promiscuity or dangerous sexual behavior
- Compulsive shopping
- Self-injury/self-mutilation
- Gambling addiction
- Sex/love addiction
- Nicotine addiction
- Internet addiction

Any of these behaviors may have been learned in childhood, or adopted as a way to cope with your own feelings of pain. Breaking them isn't easy. Each time you engage in compulsive behavior, you promise yourself that you aren't going to be a victim any longer—yet you soon find yourself running around the same patterns of behavior. If you are unable to manage a compulsive behavior, a therapist can be invaluable in helping you break the cycle. Once you know why you are compelled to act a certain way, you can begin to address the root of the problem.

> **❝** Sometimes repetition compulsion doesn't manifest itself in behaviors that appear to be unhealthy. **❞**

Real-life example: Erin's story

Sometimes repetition compulsion doesn't manifest itself in behaviors that appear to be unhealthy. Someone who is very driven might simply seem like an ambitious and confident person, when in reality the person struggles with the need to be in control at all times. This was the case for Erin, a 35-year-old vice-president at an assets management firm. Erin has always been ambitious and aggressive, and has never been afraid to pursue her desires, whether that meant moving to a new city or making the first move on a hot guy at a bar. Despite Erin's go-getter attitude, her relationships have a typical pattern—they tend to go sour around month three and end around month six. Although Erin has a cool and collected exterior, the truth is that she is tired of being alone and wants to start a family. All of her friends are coupled up, most with kids, and she wonders why that can't happen for her. She's attractive, smart, and self-assured—so, what's the problem?

Erin is ready to find out. With the help of a relationship therapist, she starts trying to identify common themes in her relationships. First, Erin and her therapist notice that she has a definite type: the artistic, brooding, sensitive guy. She often dates struggling musicians who barely earn a living. Second, they notice that Erin generally approaches and pursues a new love interest herself. Often, Erin chooses—and sometimes even pays for—the dates. As the relationship continues, Erin directs many other aspects of her boyfriend's life. Although she encourages his artistic endeavors, she often finds herself complaining to her friends and family, wondering why he can't be more aggressive and ambitious about his music career. Soon the two are fighting all the time, and they eventually break up, leaving Erin confused and heartbroken, though she doesn't show this on the outside.

As Erin and her therapist further examine her childhood, they talk about her parents' relationship. Her father ruled their home with an iron fist, while her mother played a very supporting role. Despite her passivity, she preached to her daughter that she should never depend on a man. Erin internalized this message and unconsciously took it to heart by becoming her father in her relationships. Yet while being in control helped her to feel safe, it didn't allow her partner to step up. Not only did this make him feel emasculated, it also diminished her attraction to him. She was creating her own monster, in him and the relationship.

Her therapist helped Erin to see that while she sought out men who were submissive and easygoing, she eventually became frustrated by these qualities—even though the guy was simply staying true to himself. Erin also learned that by taking the dominant role in the relationship, she was making it impossible for any man to romance her and sweep her off her feet. Her therapist assured her that it's okay to be attracted to artistic personalities, but that she should still find someone who is ambitious, hardworking, and shares similar life goals. A year later, Erin met a music producer who wasn't afraid to make the first move and could match her fiery personality. By bringing awareness to her relationship patterns, Erin was able to break out of an unhealthy cycle and find someone who could challenge and support her.

The lovemap

The habit of being attracted to the same type over and over again is known as a lovemap in the therapy world. Psychologist Dr. John Money, who pioneered the theory of lovemaps, believed that our early experiences and sexual attractions define all of our later relationships, even decades into the future.

Your relationship blueprint

A lovemap can be defined as one's blueprint for the perfect mate, both sexually and otherwise. It is the unconscious outline in your mind of what love should look like. Your lovemap is mostly the result of early childhood preferences and experiences. Much of it was absorbed before you knew what to make of it—a delicious smell, a beautiful hair color, a great sense of humor. It is a map of what is significant to you sensually, based on what resonated with you as a child.

Your lovemap is flexible until about age seven and it then solidifies in its most fundamental form. In a more informal way, however, lovemaps extend throughout your developmental years as a result of big events or relationships in your life. Your first love might set a pattern of attraction, either because it went so well or so wrong. Or, your parents' divorce and your dad's subsequent emotional departure might cause you to seek out unavailable men.

In our earlier example, if Erin had delved even deeper into her relationship patterns, she might have been able to identify why she was so attracted to artistic types. Perhaps when was younger she had a crush on a neighbor who was always playing the guitar. To go even further, perhaps Erin took the lead in her relationship with the neighbor boy, and he enjoyed her aggressive tactics. This helps explain why she then tried to be in charge in her later relationships. Her very first romantic experience mistakenly taught her that controlling others was easy, and that men need to be led.

Understanding your lovemap

Understanding your lovemap can help you to have a better relationship. When you and your partner fit together like two pieces of a puzzle, it's for a variety of reasons—both good and bad. The upside of being with someone who fits our lovemap is that we get to experience that frenzied, euphoric lust

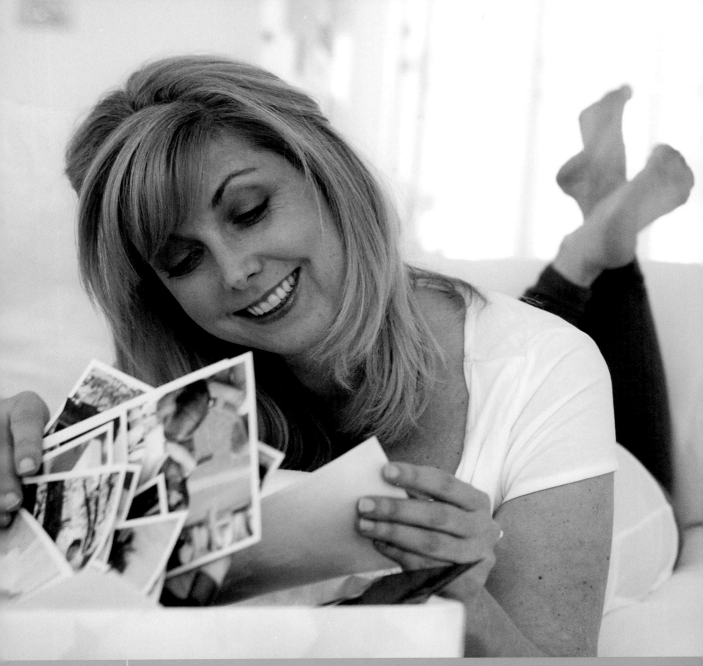

66 I deserve to find a partner who loves me, respects me, and fulfills me. 99

> **❝** Our lovemaps are why we're able to fall madly in love, only to find ourselves in a relationship tangle. **❞**

that sparks between two people who have a unique chemistry. The downside is that we may be drawn to someone who resurrects conflicts, big or small, from our childhood. It's why we're able to fall madly in love, only to find ourselves in a relationship tangle that seems impossible to manage.

The good news is that resurrecting these conflicts isn't always a bad thing if it's the right kind of personality combination. As Erin learned, there's a big difference between someone who relies on you to direct his life and someone who admires your strong personality, but seeks to challenge you. Following your lovemap is not a bad thing—in fact, in most cases it's unavoidable. What's important is to identify the major factors that have influenced your lovemap, learn what you need and expect in a relationship, and commit yourself to finding a relationship that meets your expectations and needs in a healthy way.

Since our lovemaps are formed before we even reach adulthood, they are generally born from watching the model of our parents' relationship, or from childhood crushes and societal structures. If you grew up with parents who exhibited a healthy and loving relationship, you will likely draw certain positive subconscious (and conscious) conclusions about what a relationship should look like. You will also gain very personal ideas about how men and women should treat each other, including how sexual attraction should occur in a relationship.

Vandalized lovemaps

As you can imagine, early childhood abuse (especially sexual abuse) can make for very problematic lovemaps. Dr. Money refers to these as "vandalized lovemaps," which means that early negative experiences hijacked a still-forming mind and caused it to associate pain with pleasure, or sex with trauma. For example, a young girl who was sexually molested by an older relative might find that she later craves sexual experiences with inappropriate people, such as authority figures, or that she engages in risky sex.

A good example of a vandalized lovemap at work is actually the result of something that people once considered quite harmless—childhood spanking. The Family Research Laboratory at the University of New Hampshire has released findings that link corporal punishment during childhood with sexual problems in adulthood. According to their findings, children who were punished by spanking and other methods of corporal punishment were more likely to exhibit dangerous sexual behavior in their adolescence and adulthood, including risky sex (such as promiscuous sex or sex without a condom), physical or verbal coercion for sex, and masochistic sex.

Children who grow up in punitive homes where physical and verbal abuse is utilized often suffer from poor self-esteem, which can lead them to engage in dangerous behavior—such as sex without a condom—simply because they do not respect or care about their own well-being. The fine line between spanking and physical abuse can be blurred, both in the child's mind and in the parent's mind. Additionally, little boys who are spanked over their parent's lap are receiving indirect genital stimulation, further blurring the line between pleasure and pain.

This association of pleasure and punishment also happens mentally. The child's parents, a natural source of love and support, are also inflicting pain upon the child, which creates a distorted link between love and pain. Thus, when these children grow up and engage in romantic relationships, they want to find pain where they find love—which leads them to seek masochistic interests, promiscuity, and other risky sexual behaviors. These adult behaviors help victims of abuse to normalize their childhood experiences of pain, and it gives them a false sense of control over their suffering.

Linking sex and violence

Lovemaps that link sex and violence are not uncommon. Women and men who have suffered past abuse tend to fantasize about rape and experiment with extreme forms of S & M behavior. Additionally, both women and men who were sexually abused during their childhood gravitate toward promiscuous and dangerous sexual behavior.

Escaping these early lessons of sex and violence can be difficult, especially as our bodies and our brains begin to yearn for a certain type of stimulation. Fortunately, there is nothing destructive about a little healthy sexual experimentation, whether it involves light bondage or spanking, and many partners can safely role-play these fantasies. However, a sex life that is built upon extreme pain and the abuse of power is the result of an unhealthy lovemap, and couples should be careful when implementing this type of role-play.

As you can see, lovemaps can play a distinct role in repetition compulsion. They might cause you to continually seek out mates who are abusive, unable to commit, or simply not a good match for you. They might also cause you to engage in harmful patterns or behaviors, including certain abusive sexual activities. If you notice that you are engaging in repetitive, unhealthy relationship patterns, look inward and ask yourself why you're choosing to invite certain people into your life. If you're following a blueprint of negative childhood experience, it is a good idea to seek out a counselor to help you work through these feelings and construct healthier relationship expectations.

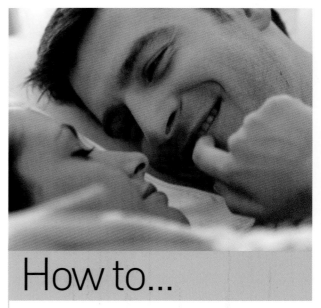

How to...

EVALUATE YOUR LOVEMAP

While it's technically impossible to "build" a lovemap, you do have the power to control your life and your relationships. If there are pieces of your lovemap that aren't working, remember that you are in charge. A healthy lovemap is about understanding any issues, facing them, and starting to work through them.

1 Ask yourself what goes wrong in your love life. Do you get involved with unavailable men? Do you suffer from feelings of abandonment? A therapist can help you get to the root of any problem areas.

2 Accept an unhappy past. You can't change it, but you can choose to allow any hurtful or negative experiences to make you stronger.

3 Move toward the future. Once you know why you are attracted to bad boys or unavailable men, you can accept your attraction without acting on it. Enjoy the attraction, then look for those feelings in a man who is available and will treat you well.

Discovering your lovemap

Learning about your own personal lovemap is important in order to understand your relationship past and direct your relationship future. To do this, think about your memories of relationships, sensuality, and attraction, starting from when you were very young. Your entire history, not just what you think of as your relationship history, contributes to your lovemap.

Lovemap construction

Sometimes a person's lovemap isn't immediately obvious, especially if you don't have a clear "type." It's easy for people who gravitate toward the same physical characteristics over and over again to notice that they have a thing for guys with tattoos or women with curly hair, but what about those who date a wide variety of people? It could be that you have an internal lovemap, and that you gravitate toward a person's personality or charisma. Reflect on the questions below in order to help track your lovemap.

What are your memories of your earliest crush?
Perhaps he was in your first grade class, he always wore a Superman t-shirt, he bullied you, or he had a lot of friends. There are a million more details you might trace. Little memories like these can help take you back to your very first feelings of attraction.

What love lessons did you learn from your parents?
Maybe you learned that marriage is about compromise. Maybe you learned that being married isn't very much fun—or even that it can be dangerous and violent. Ideally, you learned that marriage is about partnership and mutual enjoyment of each other's company. Whether your parents were best friends or constantly at odds with each other, their relationship impacted you deeply and is a major contributing factor to your lovemap.

What are the main qualities your father exhibited, both to you and to the rest of your family?
Remember how you used to think of your father when you were a child. Was he your hero, responsible for chasing away the monsters in your closet and taking you to dance class every Saturday? Did he encourage your interests and make your home somewhere you felt safe and loved? Or, was he distant and removed, always

grumpy about something that happened at the office? Your father's behavior taught you lessons about how men should act, and may have dictated what qualities you find attractive in men.

What drew you to your first love? For some, your first love might be your current partner, but for most of us, this person has long since disappeared from our lives. Think back to what made you fall in love for the first time. Don't just think generically, such as "He was smart" or "He was sweet." Think about his demeanor toward you and other women, about how he presented himself, and about how the sexual attraction was born—maybe he made you laugh, or stood up for you when no one else did, or drove a motorcycle and wasn't afraid of anything. All of these memories are part of your lovemap.

What about your next boyfriend, and the one after that? What qualities did they have in common? Think about it this way: If your exes all met in one room, would they have anything to talk about? Are they all into music? Do they all share a kooky sense of humor? The qualities they share might not be positive. For example, maybe you've dated men who are sarcastic or arrogant. Perhaps they all refused to commit to you, or made jokes that went too far. Consider all these things, positive and negative.

Think about your current partner. What does he have in common with your past loves? By now, you should start seeing a pattern among your partners. You might find that you are drawn to men who are outgoing and have a ton of friends. Along with this, however, you might find that your partners repeatedly don't make you a priority, or that they struggle with fidelity. Analyzing the good and the bad together is a critical part of defining and understanding your lovemap.

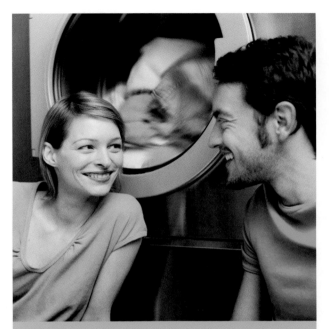

The truth about...

THE ROOTS OF ATTRACTION

In order to discover your lovemap, you have to mentally journey back in time. Think back to your first crush, or the first time you felt a strong, affectionate connection to someone outside your immediate family. Was it a teacher who was so supportive of you? The superhero you idolized? Small memories like these often hold the key to our current attraction and relationship patterns.

If you can't remember the details, talk to family or friends about memories they have of you during that time, including what interested you or who you liked spending time with. Walking down memory lane can be entertaining and useful, and can help you pinpoint the roots of your relationship patterns.

Recovering from trauma

If there are painful or abusive parts of your past that you haven't yet worked through, seeking therapy is an essential part of self-restoration. Talking openly with a therapist can help you acknowledge and identify the pain you have gone through, and restore and reclaim a healthy outlook—emotionally, relationally, and sexually.

Seeking therapy

A therapist can offer you a nonjudgmental point of view and a safe place to discuss your feelings, and to help you break unhealthy patterns and make better relationship choices. If your lovemap has roots in childhood trauma, it is especially important to speak with a therapist. Too often people assume that time heals all wounds, but this is simply not true, especially when it comes to early sexual abuse. In fact, covering up childhood abuse can be more damaging than the abuse itself, and can cause you to wonder if you imagined or even encouraged the abuse.

Many women think they have no "right" to be upset about an abusive past, especially if their current situation is mostly peaceful. However, even if you have a great job, a loving partner, a nice house, and other desirable things, that doesn't mean you

How to...

RECLAIM YOUR SEXUALITY

The best way to overcome a sexual trauma is to reclaim your sexuality for yourself. This means working to really connect with what turns you on.

1 Start building from the ground up, beginning with touching and cuddling and going from there. Sometimes certain sexual behaviors are off limits because they are associated with the trauma. All of this is totally normal and completely okay.

2 Accept that you can't rewrite your history. The only way to move on is to accept that you cannot change your past—but you can change your future.

> **"Too often people assume that time heals all wounds, but this is simply not true when it comes to abuse."**

shouldn't express sadness or anger about what happened to you—even if it was decades ago. Talking to a therapist can be invaluable, particularly if you have wounds that prevent you from fully opening up and trusting your partner. You might even find it hard to connect with your partner during sex as a result of abuse, without realizing that your past is the reason you feel hesitant to try new things or explore your sexuality.

Going to therapy can be daunting at first. That is why it is so important to find the therapist who is right for you (for more information on finding a therapist, see page 76). If you are hesitant, remember that therapy is not always the same long-term commitment that it used to be. Now, it can be short-term, lasting anywhere from a few months to a few years, depending on the issues you are working through. With the right therapist, therapy sessions can become one of the most peaceful and affirming parts of your life.

Working through conflicting emotions

Since 90 percent of sexual abuse occurs at the hands of a close friend or family member, it can cause the victim to feel very confused or guilty. Even though the abuse was not wanted, it might have caused some positive feelings. You might have felt important because the abuser told you that you were special, or perhaps he forced your silence by saying that you asked for it, causing you to believe and internalize that the abuse was your fault. Sometimes abuse can even lead to physical pleasure—after all, there is sexual touch going on, usually with someone you admire or love—which can lead to even more complicated feelings of shame or guilt.

It is important to recognize that even if you experienced some of these feelings of emotional and physical pleasure, it does not mean that the abuse was warranted or that you wanted the abuse to occur. When someone tells a child that she is special, she believes it, even if the person who is telling her this is a child abuser. And, when someone manipulates your body in a way that causes physical pleasure, you can't help but experience those good feelings.

As you can see, abuse is complicated and can cause emotional twists and turns, even for an adult. It can lead you to pick partners who are controlling and abusive, because you have been trained to associate these qualities with your first feelings of sexual pleasure and attraction. It isn't fair and it isn't right—but it happened, and until you find a way to break the hold of this sexual history, you won't be able to pick partners who respect you and care for you. For more tools to help you recover from trauma, see Resources, page 250.

While nothing can take the place of face-to-face therapy sessions, there are many good books available that can also be useful healing tools (see Resources, page 250). Talking openly with friends or family members can also help you process the reality of what happened to you, and move forward through your pain. You can also look for support groups for abuse victims in your area.

Rewriting relationship scripts

Even if you didn't experience childhood trauma, you might still be attracted to unhealthy relationships or unavailable men based on a part of your unique lovemap. Fortunately, there are ways that you can work through these obstacles, too. Follow the steps below to break out of negative patterns and change your love life for the better.

Step one: Break things off

Break off communication with the ex from hell. You know the one I am talking about: He's never there when you need him, but is always calling you late at night when he's had a few too many drinks (or vice versa). He knows he can take advantage of you because you are still vulnerable from the breakup. You still get excited by his phone call and fantasize about your relationship working someday, even though your friends and family tell you to break it off once and for all. Take their well-intentioned advice and stop answering the phone when he calls. The best way to leave the past behind is to decide not to get sucked back into hurtful scenarios by a guy who wants you for the moment, but not for forever. Remind yourself: It's his loss!

Step two: Replace bad thoughts

Be purposeful about writing down any negative thoughts and feelings. Now that you know why you are attracted to certain types, you can also start to identify the unique scripts in your head that are informing this selection. In other words, if you have a running dialogue in your head that says you are overweight, unintelligent, worthless, or any other negative quality, you aren't going to pick a partner who treats you with respect. Write down your most common negative thoughts. Think about where each thought came from and write that down, too (for example, perhaps your emotionally abusive mom often said that you were fat, or your first boyfriend called you a slut after you lost your virginity to him). Notice how many of these negative thoughts were actually implanted by others and then internalized by you as true. Are you ready to let go of them? Can you look at each belief about yourself, examine where it came from, and decide to no longer carry that voice in your head as the woman you are now?

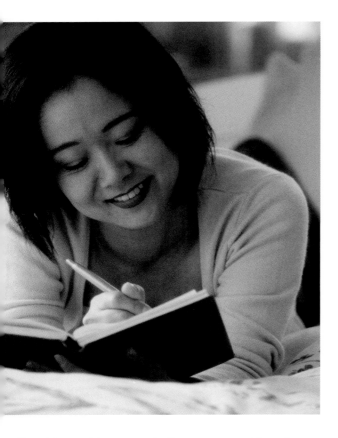

Step three: Acknowledge challenges

Notice when those negative thoughts reappear. Despite your symbolic bonfire, the truth is that negative thoughts will inevitably rear their ugly heads once in a while, especially if you are having a bad day. Don't get upset when this happens. Instead, stop, notice what is happening, accept it, and move on. For example, if you are getting dressed for a night out and you feel frustrated by how your body looks in your dress, acknowledge it. For example, "I am really beating myself up right now. It isn't likely that my body looks any different than it usually does, so there must be something else going on. Maybe I am upset because I am feeling nervous about how this date is going to go." As you acknowledge these thoughts rather than fight them, you can take control of your own mind and release the tension.

Step four: Step out of your cycle

Make new traditions. You can't let go of the past mentally if you keep returning to it physically. If you feel stuck in a cycle of bad decisions, change your routine. Try a new spot on girls' night, or volunteer at a shelter in a new part of town. You can even try taking a new route to work. By physically forcing yourself out of the same surroundings, you can start a mental shift, too. Plus, you never know who you will meet when you leave your comfort zone.

Consider making a symbolic gesture and burning or ripping up the list. As you erase the evidence of your thoughts, imagine those thoughts leaving your mind. In their stead, begin keeping a journal of affirmations (such as "I am worthy of a partner who treats me like a princess") or things you are grateful for ("I am happy I have great friends who love me"). Whenever you find yourself having negative thoughts, remember that they came from others, not from yourself, and make a conscious decision to let them go. With practice, you will find it easier and easier. You will also find that your confidence and happiness grow, along with your chances of finding a healthy, loving relationship.

> 66 Whenever you find yourself having negative thoughts, make a decision to let them go. 99

Considering relationship roles

While repetition compulsions can be very personal, some relationship patterns are especially common, and can hold many women back from being happy and fulfilled. These behavioral patterns are more exaggerated versions of the classic relationship roles of **Victim**, **Villain**, and **Hero**. Once you can identify which ones you're susceptible to, you can make a conscious effort to play a different role.

Ms. Fix-it

You may have heard women joke that they "trained" their husbands. No wonder men refer to being in the doghouse! In many ways, women treat their partners like their pets, punishing them for bad behavior and rewarding them for good behavior.

Ms. Fix-it is a classic spin-off of the **Hero** role (for more on **Hero** behavior, see pages 26–27). The problem is that there is no way to fix another person. If you try to change your partner, you risk creating serious distance between you. He is the only one who can decide to change his behavior. Don't look for a man you can model into Mr. Right. Instead, look for the real Mr. Right—trust me, he's out there.

The shape-shifter

Some women are so ready to find love that they shape-shift, assuming certain characteristics or interests that they think will please a man. For example, a woman who is bored by sports might pretend to have an interest in football. In some cases, it can go even deeper. Some women hide their sexual experience, or even change their religious beliefs or political ties to impress a man.

Shape-shifters set themselves up to be **Victims** (for more on **Victim** behavior, see pages 24–26). If you are not being real, your relationship will not feel real. Stick to the advice your mom gave you when you were embarking on your first date—be yourself. It's better than trying to impress the wrong man.

The superwoman

Many women thrive on being superheroes, often working a full-time job and also acting as CEO of their household and their relationship. However, this has created a dangerous trend that sociologists call the "double shift." Superwomen spend all day working a shift at the office and then come home to start their second shift running the home. This is

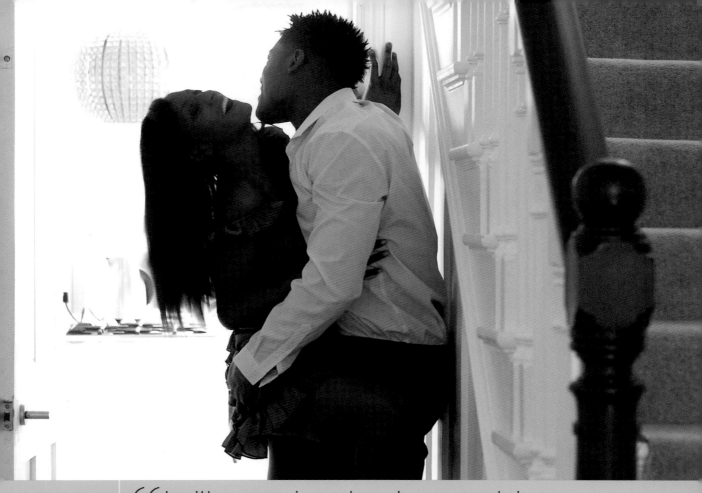

66 I will recognize when I am stuck in a
damaging role and try to shift out of it. 99

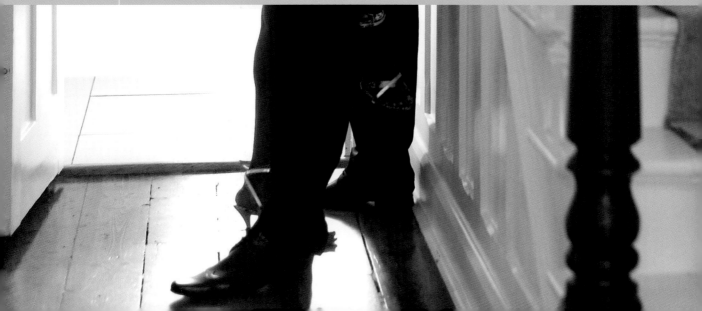

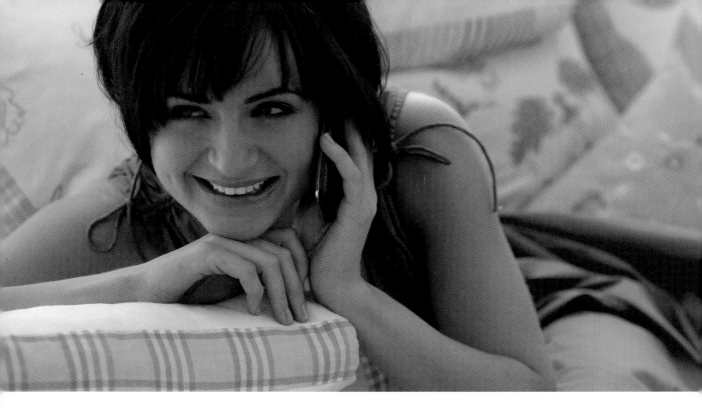

stressful, but it also comes with a gratifying feeling of power. It's great to feel needed, but the downside is that you also feel overwhelmed, unappreciated, and downright exhausted.

This is textbook **Hero** behavior, but the truth is that you can't do it all. Let your partner help you, even if he doesn't do things exactly as you would do them. Then, use that extra free time to do something truly worthwhile, like talking to the kids or relaxing in a hot bath. You'll be much happier if you enjoy your family instead of managing them.

The passive partner

If you're unhappy with your sex life and aren't initiating change, remember that no man can read a woman's mind. You must speak up and take an active role in this critical part of your relationship.

Passive partners combine the characteristics of a **Villain** and a **Victim** (for more on this, see pages 24–26). The truth is that if you want to spice up your sex life, you are the only one who can make it happen. You and your partner are responsible in

equal parts for where your sex life has landed, and you can be the one to shift it. Want romance? Light some candles and open a bottle of wine. Need more naughty in the bedroom? Buy a sex toy or a racy piece of lingerie. Breathe life into your relationship by creating a little of the excitement you crave.

Looking for the next big thing

A fact of love is that the rush of adrenaline and giddiness that comes at the start of a relationship doesn't last forever. Long-term relationships are comfortable and secure, but some women become so attached to those early feelings of excitement and lust that they struggle to stay committed and fall into the **Villain** role. No matter how caring their partner is, they can't help but wish for that new spark of passion. What they have isn't enough, because they want it all.

If you are stuck in a cycle like this, realize that the feelings of first love cannot last forever, whether you are with an average Joe or a mega celebrity. Also realize that just because the "crush" feelings have faded does not mean the passion also has to fade. Recognize and treasure the fact that with the right person, it will be replaced by a deep, sincere, and lasting commitment.

Hoping for a Hollywood happy ending

Perhaps the reason that women are often "looking for the next big thing" is because Hollywood so often promotes fictionalized expectations of love (for more on this, see page 150). Unfortunately, our patience and commitment inevitably become strained if we don't view our relationships in a realistic light. In a sense, this turns us into **Victims**, particularly when it comes to our sex lives. Real sex isn't always spontaneous or orgasmic, and most couples have to work to keep sex special and mutually pleasurable. Not every moment in your relationship will be film-worthy, but if you work at it and communicate well, your relationship will last far longer than the sparks onscreen.

Mum is the word

When it comes to communicating with our partners, the female well of words tends to dry up. We don't explain our feelings because we think our partners should be able to figure out why we're upset or sad. The truth, however, is that silence isn't effective. Worse, it turns you into a **Victim** and a **Villain**.

What is the victory in the silent treatment? There is none, and you know that—it's just hard to break the habit. However, your relationship depends on your ability to communicate. So, the next time you are mad, explain your thinking in a clear, calm way. You will be amazed at how much easier communication is when you speak up.

Metabolism maven

Poor body image is a theme that dominates many women's lives, and it can turn you into a **Victim**. Whether you constantly point out your flaws to your partner or refuse to get undressed in front of him, it can harm your relationship and your sex life. Unfortunately, unhealthy eating is perhaps the most common compulsive behavior women exhibit. This is dangerous, especially because we unintentionally pass these unsafe behaviors on to our daughters and nieces. Breaking this pattern is crucial for true physical and emotional health—and, by extension, for the health of your relationship. For more on how to do this, see pages 88–91.

Loose lips

Gossip is always a destructive force, but when it comes to private matters within your relationship, it can be devastating. Complaining to your friends about your partner is disrespectful, and has the potential to permanently harm the trust in your relationship. Because of this, it is important not to tell your friends intimate details about your relationship, even if they tell you anything and everything about their own relationships.

While it can be helpful to use a trusted friend as a sounding board, you turn into a **Villain** when you stretch things too far. Any time you are upset with your partner, the best decision is to go to your partner and talk it out. When you do this, you keep gossip from poisoning your relationship.

The perfume of desperation

Many single women fall into the trap of giving away too much too soon—not just sexually, but also in terms of time, energy, and attention. It might be a cliché, but men really do love the thrill of the chase. If you are the one to approach him, send the first text, and make the first call, you will make it seem as if your life is not already full and fulfilling.

Technology can make it easy to make frequent contact without actually making the traditional phone call. Resist the urge to forward funny emails or find him on social networking sites. Instead, let him come to you. Being centered and whole without a man will make you all the more attractive.

TOP 10 RELATIONSHIP COMMANDMENTS

Certain rules are like golden tickets for the success of your relationship. Following them can help you break out of damaging relationship patterns and rewrite your relationship blueprint. Read these rules, share them with your partner, make them part of your relationship mindset, and then vow to keep them.

1 Thou shalt not gossip about your partner.

Gossip is a destructive force in any relationship, particularly with a romantic partner. It erodes your trust and leads to miscommunication and misunderstandings. Make it a mutual rule to never, ever gossip about each other. You won't regret it.

2 Thou shalt not pretend nothing is wrong when you are upset.

Pretending that nothing is wrong is a surefire way to prolong an argument and lead to resentment and bitterness. It also keeps you from getting your needs met in the relationship, both in the moment and over the long-term.

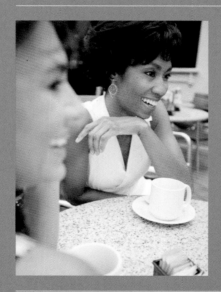

6 Thou shalt not spend your life worrying about ten pounds.

If you aren't happy with your body, you can take steps to change it. Just remember that no woman really looks like an airbrushed model. Feeling guilty about your body is a killer for your confidence and your relationship.

7 Thou shalt have realistic expectations for your love life.

Romantic comedies aren't real life! Real relationships take work—and they can even be boring and uninspired at times. It's up to you to keep the spark alive. Once you take the initiative, your partner will likely follow suit.

3 Thou shalt take control of your own sexual pleasure.

Remember that you are responsible for learning how your anatomy and sexual response work. Your partner can't make you happy if you don't tell him directly and openly what you like and don't like in the bedroom.

4 Thou shalt be hard to get, not play hard to get.

Don't pretend to be a busy, successful, happy person—be one! Stay active and challenged in other parts of your life, and romance with a respectful partner will follow. The best way to meet the right person is to become the right person.

5 Thou shalt not have a wandering eye.

Fidelity is the cornerstone of a happy relationship. There is nothing wrong with looking at and appreciating someone you find attractive, but there's never an excuse for cheating in a monogamous relationship, even if you feel your needs aren't being met.

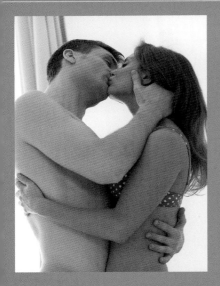 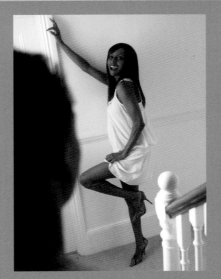 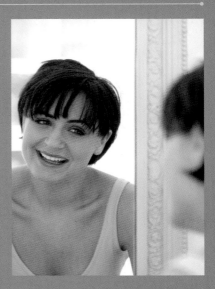

8 Thou shalt ask for help and work as a team.

You have to communicate and work together in order for your relationship to succeed. Trying to be Superwoman will leave you angry, frustrated, and disconnected from your partner. Teamwork and shared responsibility is always the best way.

9 Thou shalt not try to fix your partner.

You can work on your relationship, but you can't work on your partner. You can't change him; he has to change himself. The good news is that if you shift, he likely will, too. Inspire relationship change by looking inward and working on yourself.

10 Thou shalt be true to thine own self.

Simply put, don't try to be someone you are not. It's useless and frustrating to mimic your sister's life or your friend's relationship. Your relationship might be quite different than those of your friends or family, but that doesn't make it wrong!

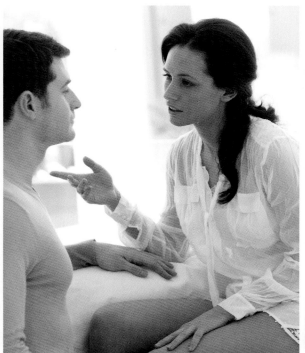
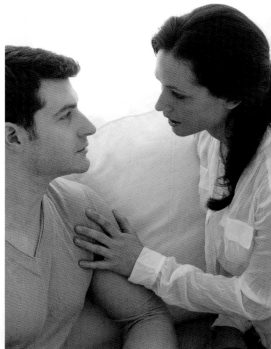

Chapter 3

When your mind feels like the enemy

Our mental landscapes can be influenced by a variety of factors: family relationships, childhood experiences, genetics, personal relationship history. For many of us, one or more of these factors can become an obstacle to finding and keeping the relationship we truly want. Identifying and treating your unique mental challenges is foundational to building a happy love life.

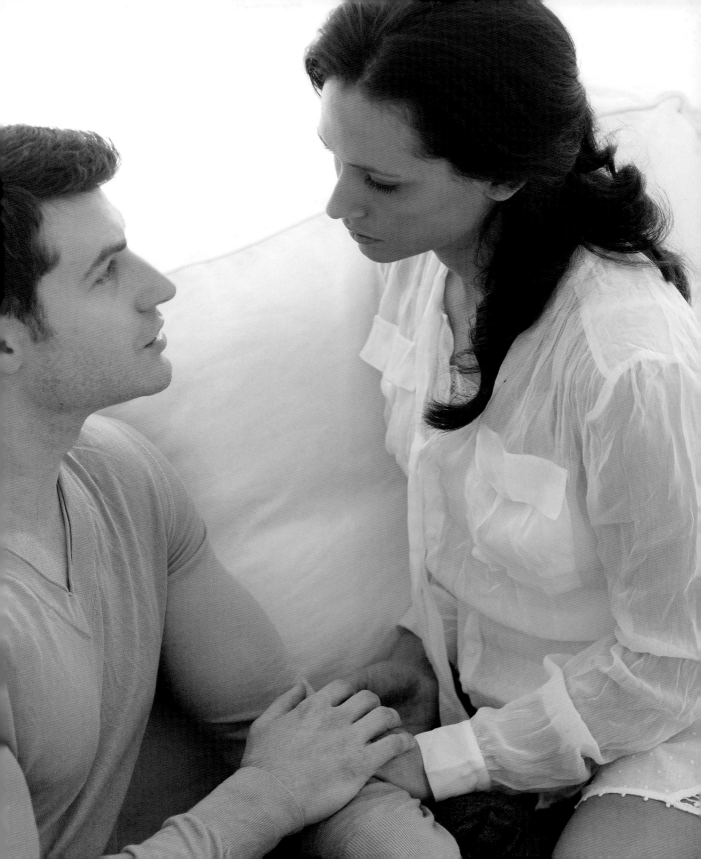

Generally speaking, no one is harder on you than you. Whether you are mentally beating yourself up for gaining five pounds or for making a mistake in a meeting, your inner monologue is often very negative. Worse, it doesn't matter how well you rebound from your mistakes—for most women, external changes like these can't allay feelings of guilt or low self-worth. The only way to bring equanimity to your mind is to make internal changes.

The topics covered in this chapter will help you identify where you need to make these internal shifts. To start, be brutally honest with yourself as you take this quiz. Your answers will help you detect any potentially negative thought processes.

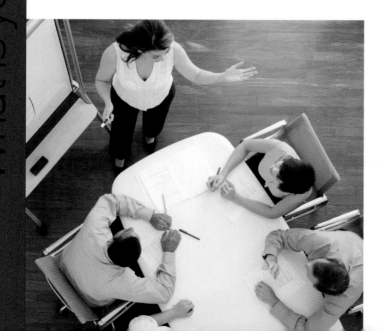

1 YOUR LONG-AWAITED DATE NIGHT IS HERE AT LAST

As you get ready for a night out with your partner, what thoughts are going through your head?

A I hope he doesn't expect any action tonight. I didn't make it to the gym once this week and I am sure he will not find me sexy!

B I can't wait to finally have some romantic time without the kids.

C The babysitter is going to be upset about how wound up the kids are. Maybe I should just cancel the date and stay home?

2 YOU HAVE A BIG PRESENTATION

to give to your executive board. On the way to work, all you can think is:

A No matter what I do, my boss is going to find something wrong with my work and won't give me that raise I have been expecting. She is so critical.

B This is my shot to show my boss what I am made of!

C I feel bad taking this presentation when my co-worker really wanted this opportunity. I hope she isn't mad at me. Maybe I should have turned it down.

3 YOU ARE HANGING OUT WITH YOUR GIRLFRIENDS

for some much needed R & R. One of your friends (who is known for being very direct) makes a snarky comment about your parenting skills. You:

A Laugh it off uncomfortably and then spend the next few weeks fuming miserably and talking badly about her to the rest of your friends.

B Smile sweetly and say, "That's a little hurtful. I don't think that I quite understand why you would say that."

C Immediately start crying and spend the rest of the night being comforted.

4 YOUR PARTNER VOLUNTEERS TO WATCH THE KIDS

and do the dishes after dinner, so that you can take a hot bath and relax. You say:

A "I think it will be easier for me to do this myself. Last time you watched the kids alone, they left a huge mess that took hours to clean up."

B "Only if you promise to join me in the tub once the kids are in bed!"

C "Don't be silly. I am not tired at all! Doing the dishes gives me time to unwind and reflect on my day."

5 YOU AND YOUR PARTNER HAVE A ROMANTIC NIGHT

that ends in intimacy. He rushes through foreplay and you end up unsatisfied. What do you do?

A Roll your eyes in the dark of the bedroom and call your girlfriend the next day to whine about his uninspiring lovemaking skills.

B Ask him if he wants to go again and if not, request that he do a little "afterplay" on you.

C Fake an orgasm and then roll over and go to sleep.

6 WHEN WEIGHING YOURSELF AT THE GYM YOU NOTICE

that you have gained five pounds since you last checked two weeks ago. You:

A Feel stressed and angry that you aren't able to control this part of your life, and vow to cut all carbs and sugar from your diet immediately.

B Decide to switch to working out in the morning, so your frequent after-work commitments don't interfere with your gym time so often, then call a friend and ask if she'd like to meet up for 7 AM yoga the next day.

C Immediately regret all the holiday dinner parties you and your partner have been attending. How are you supposed to lose weight when you have no control over how many calories are placed in front of you six nights out of seven?

7 YOU HAVE RECENTLY GONE THROUGH A BREAK-UP

with a man that you really thought could be "the one." How do you move on from this experience and heal?

A Complain about your ex to all of your friends. The more you think about his negative traits, the better you feel.

B Allow yourself time to be sad, but make sure you have plenty of events on your calendar to keep you active.

C Blame yourself for the break-up, wondering what it is about you that causes all men to eventually leave.

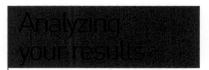

Analyzing your results

A-type answers mean that you might have some unresolved anger and blame problems. Instead of being open and honest about how you feel, most of the time you bottle up your emotions and feel frustrated or mistreated as a result. At other times, all that pent-up frustration causes you to explode or lash out at the people you love.

B-type answers indicate that you are in a healthy mental place. You know when to ask for help and how to express your needs to those around you. You have a positive attitude overall and an optimistic outlook about your relationship, your family, and your job.

C-type answers suggest that you are stuck in a people-pleasing routine that often spirals into self-blame. In addition to not being fully honest about how you feel, you frequently adopt a martyr persona, putting other people's priorities first and then blaming them for your own unhappiness. Acting this way can greatly damage your outlook and your self-esteem.

❝ The only way to bring equanamity to your mind is to make important internal changes. **❞**

Codependency

One of the things that can stand in our way of finding and keeping love is codependent behavior. Essentially, people who suffer from codependency issues struggle with the desire to fulfill all of their partner's needs, all of the time. This means that their own needs are never voiced, creating a relationship that is unbalanced and unhealthy.

What is codependency?

The concept of codependency is often misunderstood. Most people believe that someone who is codependent is someone who is needy, hates to be alone, and always has to be in a relationship. Although this is the more modern understanding of the word, the clinical definition is actually quite different.

Codependency was a term originally used in the therapy world to describe the enabling behavior of a relative of an alcoholic. However, the definition of codependency has clinically evolved to include someone who gives attention, time, comfort, money, or any other means of support to any type of addict, thereby assisting the addiction. Although the codependent has good intentions and truly wants the addict to become sober, this type of behavior is counterproductive to recovery. In reality, any assistance the codependent gives simply allows the addict to continue down a path of destruction.

While it is unknown how codependency begins, many therapists believe that it is the result of a dysfunctional childhood. If a child grows up in a home where her needs are rarely met, she will learn to deny her own emotions. This is especially true in homes where sadness and anger are considered to be negative. The child learns to deny her feelings and "play" at being happy, even when she is anxious or upset. She grows up to be a people-pleaser who can't even be honest with her own partner, which can be devastating to her happiness. For more on the characteristics of codependency, see Appendix, page 240.

Codependency and love

When we define ourselves through our ability to make those we love happy, what we are really doing is trying to make ourselves safe. In other words, our subconscious imagines that if we don't make others angry, don't rock the boat, and meet everyone else's needs, then we won't be abandoned.

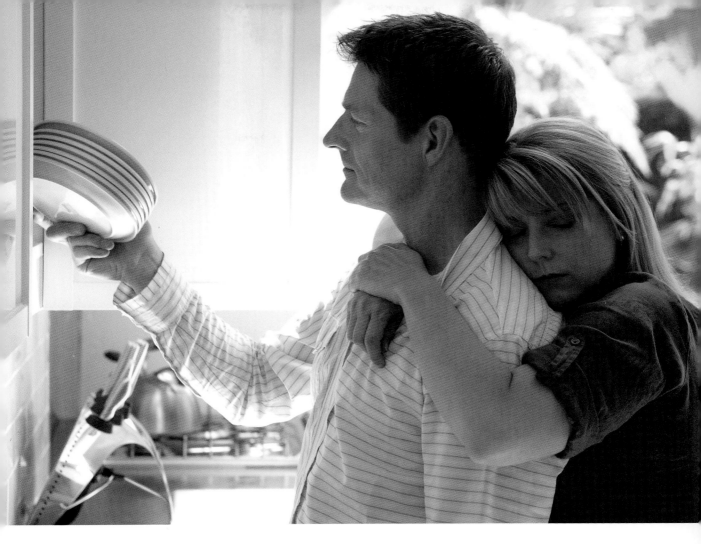

Most codependents grew up in a household where their needs weren't met, which meant that emotional or literal abandonment was a real concern. This is why it is common for people with addicted or alcoholic parents to exhibit codependent behavior. In order to safeguard against the threat of abandonment, codependents go above and beyond to ensure they are needed in the lives of those around them. Their mindset is "How can he leave me if I do everything for him and meet all of his physical and emotional needs?" Codependents imagine that if they are "good enough," "attentive enough," or "loving enough," their partner will provide the safety they crave.

There's one main reason that this type of behavior (however well-intentioned) doesn't work: If you are codependent, you are operating in the relationship from a place of fear. You are so focused on holding on to the relationship that you don't realize how guarded and insecure you really feel. This means that you won't be able to trust or truly open up in a relationship. At the same time, a codependent person eventually begins to resent her partner for failing to notice her selfless behavior. This causes her to feel victimized, and further ensures that no partner will be able to meet her needs. Ultimately, you aren't able to get the love you really want when you are trapped by codependency and fear.

When you stay in a relationship out of fear rather than by choice, you can't ask for what you need. You can't fully be your authentic self, and you are never in an empowered position. It is only when you proactively choose, every single day, to be in your relationship that you are able to build an authentic, mutually loving partnership with someone else.

Codependency outside of romantic relationships

Codependent behavior isn't just relegated to romantic relationships. People can also exhibit codependent behavior with their friends, with coworkers, or with family members. In fact, people with codependency issues usually exhibit this type of behavior with everyone in their lives.

Codependent behavior can also be complicated by the fact that codependent people tend to attract "needy" people. A codependent feels most comfortable when she is playing the role of **Hero** (for more on

this type of behavior, see pages 26–27), which attracts people who prefer to play the role of **Victim** (for more on this, see page 26). When someone with hero behavior loves or befriends someone with victim behavior, it might seem like the perfect match. The victim always needs attention, while the hero always needs to feel helpful and in control.

For a while, the hero can continue to put her focus on other people rather than herself, and the victim can continue to avoid responsibility for his or her actions. However, these relationships often quickly unravel and ultimately end in resentment because neither party is being honest about their needs or taking control of their lives.

The dangers of codependency

Codependency is tricky to diagnose because, at first glance, several of its behaviors seem positive. After all, what's wrong with trying to make other people happy or putting other people first? The

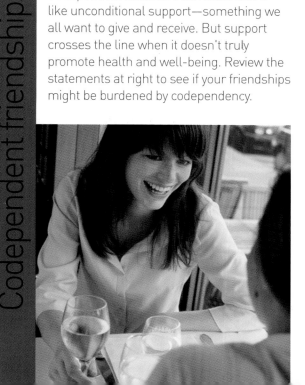

Codependent friendships

Codependent behaviors can often seem like unconditional support—something we all want to give and receive. But support crosses the line when it doesn't truly promote health and well-being. Review the statements at right to see if your friendships might be burdened by codependency.

Codependent thinking

- My feelings about myself stem from your approval.
- My mental attention is focused on protecting you.
- My self-esteem is strengthened by finding a solution to your problems.
- I spend most of my time sharing and participating in your hobbies and interests.
- I am not aware of what I want, but instead focus on what you want.
- My future dreams revolve around you.
- My fear of rejection or inciting anger influences my actions and words.
- I value your opinion more than my own.

If you find yourself identifying with a number of these statements, it is time to explore just how deep your codependency runs. A therapist can provide valuable help and counseling as you go through this process.

> **❝**Codependency is an extreme example of what can happen when people don't put their own needs first.**❞**

answer is that nothing is wrong with this—in small doses. However, too often women put answering their needs at the bottom of their to-do list, allowing everyone else's needs to come before their own. Unfortunately, this won't make you a great mom or partner. Instead, it will make you tired, frustrated, and angry. When you give all of your energy to everyone else, you have nothing left to give to the most important person in your life—you!

Codependent behavior is an extreme example of what can happen when people lose an ability to put their own needs first. Eventually, a codependent might struggle to identify what her own needs are because she is so out of touch with herself. Worst of all, codependents continually feel mistreated by those they love the most. Since they never express their own emotions or needs, they are left feeling empty, neglected, and often worthless.

If you are codependent, you might wonder why you are always giving and never receiving. You may feel as though you have the weight of the world on your shoulders, but receive no recognition for your efforts. Over time, your mental landscape will become bleak. You will start to feel as though it's you against the world, and those closest to you (your friends, your partner, your kids) become part of the problem because they don't realize how much they are draining you of your energy and happiness.

Overcoming codependency

Treating codependency can take time. In fact, codependent behaviors and thought processes might be so ingrained that counseling is required in order to fully work through your past and present struggles. Books, support groups, and one-on-one therapy are all good outlets that can help you identify and treat the codependency issues that are specific to you and proactively move forward (for more information see Resources, page 250).

In addition, one of the most effective ways to overcome codependency is to spend time alone. This is crucial, especially if you are healing from a divorce or the recent breakup of a relationship where you were a codependent partner. Resist the urge to slip back into a relationship immediately, and commit to staying single for a period of time. Whether or not you choose to heal through therapy, it is important to spend some time regrouping and getting reacquainted with yourself and your needs. If you look at how this past relationship reflects a pattern in your life, think about where and why those hurts started, and focus on healing, you will feel more empowered, and your next relationship will be much more likely to be mutually loving, authentic, and respectful.

Follow this rule of thumb: After a breakup, take a hiatus in commitment that lasts half the time of your relationship (up to four years). In other words, if your relationship was three years, remain single for at least a year and a half. If it was a six-year relationship, don't commit until three years have passed. Any relationship that lasted longer than eight years should require a minimum of four years alone for true healing to occur. This doesn't mean that you can't date or have a partner, but it means that you shouldn't make any serious commitments—such as moving in together, getting engaged, or marrying—until this period of healing has passed.

Obsessive-compulsive disorder

People often joke about this personality disorder, describing a certain behavioral quirk as their "OCD" acting up. And, to some degree, we all participate in a version of OCD behavior. Obsessive-compulsive disorder is when a person assuages an uncomfortable thought or feeling (the obsession) by engaging in a certain behavior (the compulsion).

The OCD spectrum

There are varying levels of OCD. On the less severe end of the spectrum, you may be the type who must get the dishes washed before you can relax. At a more intense level, you might feel compelled to check that the stove is off, even though you've checked it a few minutes prior. Or, you might check the locks twice each night before you go to bed.

Clinically speaking, therapists do not consider these common symptoms to be OCD behavior because they do not interfere with a person's life. People who fall under the clinical definition of OCD might find that they have difficulty leaving the house because they spend hours on routines, from hand-washing to straightening things to various other behavioral idiosyncrasies. Known as rituals, these behaviors are usually born out of a person's desire to try to control his or her life in a seemingly chaotic world. Rituals create a false sense of safety and control that can help assuage a person's anxiety, but they can make even simple things like going on a date seem impossible. For a list of OCD symptoms, see Appendix, pages 240–241.

OCD in relationships

OCD behavior almost always has a negative impact on a person's intimacy in relationships. If you suffer from this condition, you might have a hard time enjoying anything, including sex, because your brain isn't able to stop multitasking. You might regularly be too distracted to reach orgasm. Perhaps you refuse to cuddle and bask in the post-sex glow with your partner because you want to hop into the shower and "get clean." The truth is, it's impossible to be present with your partner and fully involved in your relationship when obsessive thoughts are ruling your mind. This can be confusing for your partner, who will wonder why you seem so disconnected and uninterested in his advances.

Obsessing over love

In addition to distracting from intimacy, OCD behavior can also lead to an unhealthy obsession with love. In other words, instead of obsessing about cleaning your house, you might obsess about meeting "the one," or having the perfect relationship. This is not surprising considering the hormones and brain chemicals that are released during the infatuation stage of a relationship. While feelings of intense attraction and passion are normal and even healthy in the beginning of a relationship, it is important to identify when those behaviors become obsessive and unhealthy. Brain research has shown that when one is newly in love, the dopamine center of the brain—the part largely responsible for addiction—is extremely active. So, new love is like an addiction for all of us. However, people who suffer from OCD can become obsessed with love, abandoning friendships and interests to invest 110 percent in their relationship. They make that new person the entire focus of their life, much like addicts do with their drug of choice.

When you do this, you lose sight of your identity, which almost always leads to volatile connections and unhealthy relationships. This means that it is likely that a breakup will occur. When it does, you will be left feeling shattered, and may even experience withdrawal symptoms, similar to those that substance addicts experience.

Rather than investing all your time in a new relationship, it is important that you save emotional energy for yourself and the other people in your life. Even more important, remember that no one person can complete you. You are already whole just as you are. This realization is essential to your happiness and stability, whether you are single or in a relationship. (For tips on how to create a healthy relationship and maintain appropriate boundaries and priorities, see pages 113–115.)

> **66** It's impossible to be present with your partner when obsessive thoughts are ruling your mind. **99**

Identifying and treating OCD

OCD behavior can be difficult to detect because many of its characteristics are seen as positive. This is especially true for people who have Type A personalities, and thus often naturally exhibit many OCD-like thoughts and behaviors. If you have a Type A personality, you are a perfectionist who likes everything to be "just so." You aren't the type to go to bed if the house is dirty. And, like those who suffer from OCD, Type As also typically have a harder time reaching orgasm, since this requires being present in the moment and releasing control. Type A isn't a personality disorder, but it can negatively affect your mood and your relationship.

On the outside, it seems as though Type As have everything together, which makes it hard for others to see when their behavior is veering into dangerous OCD territory. Learning how to manage stress and live in the moment can help to lessen the effects of obsessive-compulsive thoughts and behavior. If you feel unable to do this, it is a good idea to seek professional help.

Although OCD can be a devastating disorder, treatment can greatly alleviate your symptoms and help you get your life back on track. Cognitive behavioral therapy and medication can help you loosen the grip of obsessive thoughts and return to a peaceful state of mind.

Depression

Everyone has suffered from a bad case of the blues at one point or another, but sometimes feelings of sadness and defeat can actually be signs of a more serious condition, called major depressive disorder. This clinical type of depression can happen to anyone, even successful people with happy lives and strong, fulfilling relationships.

Diagnosing depression

One of the main things that sets true depression apart from other sad feelings is that the depression does not go away, even during times when you would normally feel happy. If activities that you usually enjoy leave you feeling empty, you could be experiencing more than a temporary sadness. Depression often causes you to cease doing the things you love and retreat into yourself, away from the friends and family who want to offer you support. This is the start of a vicious cycle—moving away from your support system makes you more depressed, which in turn makes you more distant, and on and on. Monitoring the things that make you feel sad and your detachment from your support group is a good way to determine whether your condition might be clinical. For more symptoms of depression, see Appendix, page 241.

Depression and love

Depression doesn't just affect how you feel; it also impacts the way people treat you and the types of relationships you create. When you are depressed, part or all of you is shut off from the world, both emotionally and physically. You don't seem approachable or friendly, and your entire body sends off the signal "Stay away!" or "I'm not available." Worst of all, you will likely attract people who are in a similarly negative frame of mind, which will only exacerbate your depression and make it harder to seek treatment.

If you are already in a relationship, depression can wreak havoc on your bond with your partner. You might find yourself snapping at your partner for no reason, or being unresponsive to his attempts to cheer you up. A relationship cannot thrive in these conditions. Over time, your partner will likely give up in exasperation, and the two of you will end up completely disconnected.

Treating depression

Symptoms of depression can quickly spiral into dangerous territory. If you are to the point where you are fantasizing about suicide or harming yourself or others, then you should speak to your doctor immediately. When seeking treatment, remember that there is no substitute for a mental health professional. It is tempting to simply talk to your medical practitioner about your feelings, but while he or she can prescribe medication, this type of doctor won't be as well-versed as a therapist in examining the roots of your depression. Don't be ashamed or embarrassed to seek the help of a therapist, as well as that of a psychiatrist, who can give a medical diagnosis and explore medical treatment. Depression is often chemical or can become chemical, meaning that it is most effective to include medication in your treatment—sometimes for just a limited time, and sometimes for much longer periods. Regardless of the length of time, medical treatment is not something to fear. Research has clearly shown that the combination of talk therapy and medication works most effectively in treating depression.

Investigate your medication options carefully. SSRIs, or selective serotonin reuptake inhibitors, can help increase the serotonin level in the brain, but it can also decrease your libido and make you less interested in intimacy. Fortunately, there are other options. Wellbutrin, a pill that has buproprion as the active ingredient, can successfully treat depression, and has been shown to have less of an impact on desire. Studies on Wellbutrin and its impact on libido are still underway, but you can speak to your doctor to see if you are a candidate for this medication. Additionally, Viagra has been shown to improve sexual response in men and women who might be experiencing sexual function concerns due to depression and medication.

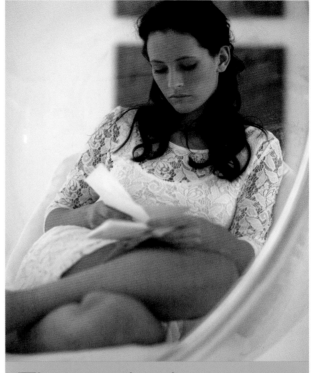

The truth about...

BATTLING LOW SELF-ESTEEM

True depression is not something that can be overcome by a strong will and a conviction to change. You need therapy and possibly medication to effectively fight this disease. However, as part of your treatment, you can choose to stop negative thoughts as much as possible. Identify the things that often make you feel sad or angry. Think about where these thoughts may have begun, then do your best to banish and replace each thought with something more positive. For more on how to do this, see pages 78–81.

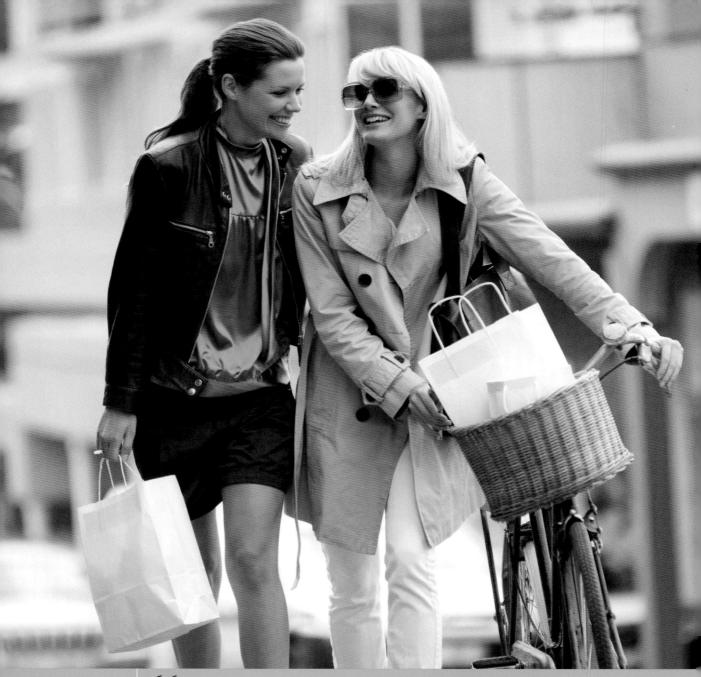

"Even when I am feeling down, I will stay active and seek to connect with others."

> **66** Research on happiness has shown that altruism is a key factor in predicting one's happiness. **99**

Lifestyle changes to treat depression

In addition to medication and therapy, there are changes you can make to your lifestyle to help heal from major depressive disorder. These lifestyle adjustments can also be a good starting point if you are experiencing occasional periods of sadness that do not fit the clinical definition of depression. No matter how mild or severe your depression, the biggest tip is this: Resist the urge to mope at home on the couch as much as possible. Although it feels comforting to retreat under the blankets with a pint of ice cream, you will only exacerbate your feelings of boredom and helplessness. Accomplishment and activity are the keys to overcoming sadness and feeling more and more like your true self.

Instead, try to stay active through exercise, spending time with friends, and getting involved in your community. Research on happiness has shown that altruism is a key factor in predicting one's happiness. One random act of kindness each week will not only make your world a better place, it will help you feel more empowered, proud, and proactive—all of which can go a long way toward combating depression and sadness. In fact, the smallest changes in routine are often the things that bring us the most joy, so following the suggestions below can be hugely healing.

Make it a point to go the gym, or get active by taking a walk with a friend or going for a swim or a bike ride. The endorphins that are released in our brain during exercise can help to combat stress and depression. They will also help you strengthen your body and feel empowered and healthy.

Examine your lifestyle. Low self-worth can cause you to neglect personal hygiene, but this only makes feelings of depression worse. While you can't find happiness at the hair salon, you can improve your self-esteem and feel more like yourself when you invest time and effort into how you look. Taking pride in your appearance cannot help but lead to an increased pride in your overall sense of self.

Talk about your feelings with your friends. Almost everyone has experienced mild depression at some point in her life, and talking about what you are going through can help you realize that you aren't alone. Be purposeful about not isolating yourself when you are feeling sad.

Give back to your community by volunteering. It can be hard to get motivated to volunteer when you are struggling with depression, so start off with small commitments, or make a pact with a friend who also wants to volunteer and will help you stay committed. Volunteer at places where your talents can really shine through, whether that's mentoring children, planning a game night at a retirement home, or spending time at your local animal shelter.

Keep a gratitude journal. It might feel a little forced at first, especially since depression makes you feel like there is little to be happy about. However, sitting down and examining the good things in your life will help you find ways to be thankful, whether it is for good friends, your cozy apartment, your sense of humor, your pet, or other little things that are uniquely yours.

Anxiety

Everyone suffers from anxiety at certain times. For some people, going on a date can cause them to be very anxious. Other people get anxious at the thought of public speaking, meeting the in-laws, or going to a party. A small amount of anxiety is normal and even healthy, but when anxiety levels become unmanageable and interfere with your daily life, then you might be suffering from an anxiety disorder.

Types of anxiety disorders

The two most common types of clinical anxiety disorders are generalized anxiety disorder and social anxiety disorder. People with generalized anxiety disorder are often overwhelmed with feelings of fear and nervousness. Those who suffer from social anxiety disorder feel nervous specifically in social situations, and might be unwilling to leave the house or interact with people.

People diagnosed with generalized anxiety disorder find that anxiety rules their lives, and might struggle with concentrating at work or sleeping as a result. Their constant worry might disrupt their career goals, or make it hard to connect with family and friends. It can also have a number of uncomfortable physical symptoms, including nausea, diarrhea, edginess or restlessness, fatigue, or difficulty falling or staying asleep. Anxiety disorders can also cause people to shut down sexually or feel unable to let down defenses with a partner. For more symptoms of anxiety disorders, see Appendix, page 241.

Anxiety in relationships

Anxiety limits the adventures we take and keeps us from experiencing life to the fullest. Some people experience anxiety around sex, especially if they have low libido. You might worry about being rejected, and feel reluctant to try new things sexually. This can cause you to shut down during sex and become disconnected from your partner.

Outside of the bedroom, your anxiety may force your partner to be fully responsible for the activities that you are too anxious to perform, such as driving the kids to school, going to the grocery store, or talking to the plumber about house repairs. This will force your partner to go into a caregiver mode, which can harm your relationship, both sexually and otherwise (see pages 104–105 to learn more about the effects of a caregiver relationship).

Treating anxiety disorders

To start, see a psychiatrist for a proper evaluation and medical diagnosis. Treatment for generalized anxiety disorder often includes cognitive behavioral therapy (CBT), in which people learn coping skills for managing anxiety. Lifestyle changes such as cutting back on caffeine, exercising, and maintaining a healthy diet can help curb stress. In some cases, medications such as benzodiazepines, buspirone, and anti-depressants are used to help treat anxiety symptoms. Although medication can be beneficial, therapy and other coping strategies are the preferred way to treat long-term anxiety, especially as some medications can be habit-forming.

Similarly, people with social anxiety generally find cognitive behavioral therapy to be helpful. A therapist can help you work through a situation that provokes anxiety, whether that is going to the store,

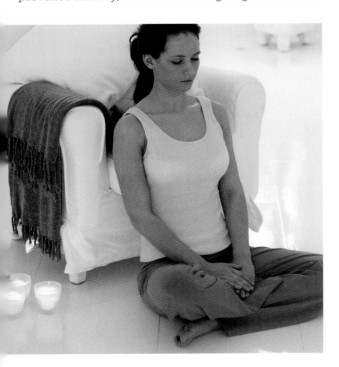

eating in public, or meeting people for the first time. Additionally, some medications (including the benzodiazepines mentioned above, as well as SSRIs and beta blockers, a class of drugs used to treat cardiac concerns) can be used to help treat the symptoms of social anxiety disorder.

Letting go of anxiety

In addition to therapy, one of the best ways to cope with anxiety—whether or not you have a diagnosed clinical disorder—is to accept the anxiety rather than judge it. Criticizing yourself for feeling anxious will not help. Instead, simply think, "I am very anxious right now. It is uncomfortable, but I know it will eventually pass." Try to identify where your anxiety level is on a scale of 1–10, and allow yourself to feel whatever emotions are sweeping over you.

Remember that anxiety is a natural human reaction, which can sometimes be advantageous. That boost of adrenaline and rush of nerves can be useful in situations that are dangerous or that require an elevated performance. Your body is trained to respond to these biological cues—and it is also trained to respond to self-soothing. Try lighting a scented candle with hints of lavender, which is shown to be relaxing. Read passages from a favorite book, or meditate quietly. Notice that your anxiety helps you be more compassionate toward others who are also anxious. All of these thoughts can help episodes of anxiety to pass.

In truth, you can never completely rid your life of anxiety. However, you can remember that you and your anxiety are separate entities. The case for this is simple: When you have a stomachache, you don't allow the physical symptoms to affect your identity. Treat your anxiety in the same way—as a painful part of life that lasts only for short periods. Continue taking part in normal activities, and remember that your anxiety doesn't rule your life—you do.

Eating disorders

Eating disorders can take on very different shapes. Some people abuse laxatives or diet pills, others starve themselves for days, only to go on a binge and eat thousands of calories in one sitting. Still others exercise for hours at a time, pushing their body past its breaking point in order to achieve weight loss.

Body image and the media

Are you happy with your body? If you have read a magazine or watched television lately, you probably aren't. Media images have an enormous impact on the way women view themselves. In fact, a recent study in the United Kingdom found that watching celebrity girl groups in music videos for even a short 10-minute period significantly decreased the average girl's self-image.

Unfortunately, escaping the media in today's society is virtually impossible. Women are constantly bombarded with billboards featuring ultra-thin models, or magazines featuring women who lost all their baby weight within the first 10 weeks of giving birth. No wonder almost 10 million women and girls and one million men and boys in the United States suffer from anorexia and/or bulimia, the two most common eating disorders worldwide.

Even worse than simply promoting slim figures, celebrity magazines routinely point out flaws in stars—generally female stars—and even go so far as to name the "best" and "worst" beach bodies each year. With magazines such as these on the shelves, it is no wonder that 81 percent of 10-year-old girls are afraid of being fat. This fear doesn't go away with maturity. From diet pills to "cleansing" fasts, many women will do anything to fit into a size two, regardless of their age or body type. As a reflection of this, statistics around eating disorders are getting consistently worse: The number of people suffering from eating disorders in the US has doubled in the last five years. For a list of symptoms of eating disorders, see Appendix, page 241.

Body image and relationships

A poor body image can greatly affect your ability to find and maintain a loving relationship. Not only will you waste valuable time feeling poorly about yourself, but you will also cut yourself off from real love and acceptance. If you can't love and accept your body, you are unlikely to find someone else who can. If you go out for a date but can't enjoy yourself because you feel uncomfortable in your dress, that lack of confidence is going to come through—especially when you only allow yourself to order a small salad and pass on dessert.

Poor body image can also affect your sexual appetite and habits. Women who do not feel confident in their bodies generally don't feel comfortable undressing in front of their partners, and may even refuse to have sex in certain positions for fear of looking flabby. In addition, crash dieting can have extremely negative effects on estrogen and testosterone levels, which will affect everything from your mood to your libido to your menstrual cycle. The bottom line is that obsessing over your weight can make you very lonely indeed.

Treating eating disorders

Ultimately, eating disorders are not about losing weight or counting calories. They are about a person's need to assert control in order to help combat the fear of living in an uncertain world. Treatment for eating disorders should be multi-faceted, as the disease itself is so complicated.

People who are suffering from an eating disorder almost always require professional help in order for true psychological and physical healing to occur. Rehabilitation and therapy are a must. A good first step is to find an individual therapist who specializes in this area of treatment. There are also 12-step groups for women who suffer from eating disorders, which can provide valuable group support during this difficult time, as well as in-patient and out-patient centers that can help. Support from your loved ones is also crucial. Antidepressants or other medications can also help if you are suffering from depression or anxiety.

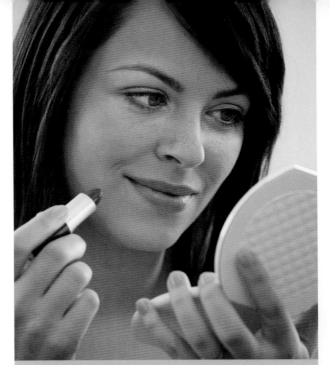

How to...

RETHINK YOUR BODY IMAGE

Just like any other part of your self-image, the way you think and feel about your body is a choice—and it is something that you can control. For women, especially, it can be very difficult to keep thoughts about the body positive. Following these steps can help you learn to love and appreciate your body.

1 Identify your best assets, then play them up. Maybe you have bright eyes or a brilliant smile. Maybe your legs go on for miles, or you have charming freckles. There are a million little things that make your own beauty uniquely alluring.

2 Build a beauty routine that you are proud of. Taking good care of your skin, hair, and body helps you connect with and enjoy your body.

3 Notice how outer beauty is colored by what's inside. Show regular kindness and strength and you will see people naturally gravitate toward you.

Disordered eating

Even if you do not fit the clinical diagnosis for an eating disorder, your body image has probably negatively affected your life at one point or another. Maybe you avoid the beach, maybe you stay in on Saturday nights, or maybe you are afraid to disrobe in front of your spouse. In an attempt to lose weight, you might embark on restrictive diets (no carbs, no white foods, no eating past 6:00 PM), or you might develop very ritualized eating patterns (eating only from a certain plate, extending meal time by chewing very slowly, indulging in a weekly "cheat day" in which your eating habits are wild and out of control).

These are signs of disordered eating, and nearly three out of four American women participate in these habits. Unfortunately, many symptoms of disordered eating are now considered quite normal. Most women would think nothing of it if a friend said she wasn't eating carbohydrates anymore, or if her mother mentioned she was going on a fruit and veggie fast. Society practically shouts at us that there's absolutely nothing wrong with wanting to lose weight, no matter what your size or shape.

The truth about...
THE NUMBERS OF WEIGHT LOSS

Exactly how many women struggle with body image? A study conducted by *Self* magazine found that 67 percent of women (excluding those with actual eating disorders) are trying to lose weight, 13 percent smoke to lose weight, 37 percent regularly skip meals to try to lose weight, and 27 percent would be "extremely upset" if they gained just five pounds. The women in this survey came from all walks of life and spanned a range of ages and ethnicities, yet they had one thing in common: they all wanted the "perfect" body.

In reality, losing weight is healthy only if you are legitimately overweight and are choosing safe methods of weight loss. However, research has found that 53 percent of dieters are already at a healthy weight and are still trying to lose weight. Moreover, many women are choosing to lose weight through restrictive or dangerous diets, or through expensive diet supplements.

Ending the "thin" epidemic

Most women already know that the best way to be healthy and maintain an appropriate weight is to eat healthy, balanced meals and to exercise regularly. Logically, you also know that you are "supposed" to love your body—but how can you embrace it when you perceive it as being riddled with flaws? One way to help yourself stop focusing on these perceived flaws is to consider the message you are sending to the young girls in your life—your daughter, your niece, or even your granddaughter. Every time you skip a meal or lament about your "fat hips" in front of your daughter you are sending her the message that your body—and therefore her body, and the female body in general—is flawed.

The only real person who can put an end to this "thin is in" epidemic is you. Ditch the diet soda cans in your fridge and replace them with natural fruits and vegetables. Avoid pre-packaged salads from fast food places and prepare a truly nutritious meal with your family. When you go to the grocery store, don't pore over the latest celebrity gossip magazines—and don't let your daughter do this either. Remind your daughter (and yourself) that all magazines airbrush their models, and then give her real heroes to look up to, starting with yourself.

Finally, don't forget the importance of exercise. Exercise helps the body function properly, and it also helps boost your mood and your self-esteem. Just one workout session can leave you feeling stronger and more confident, so incorporate this into your routine as much as possible.

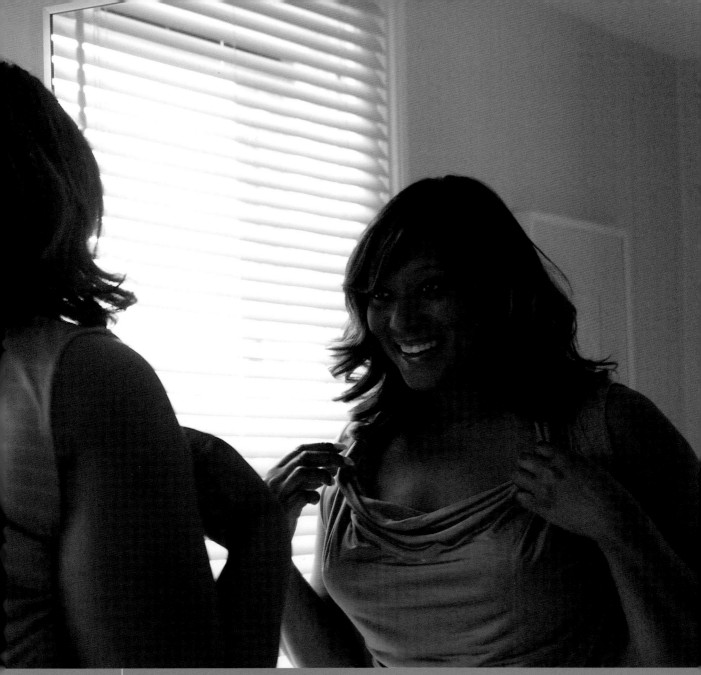

PERSONAL AFFIRMATION 66 My body turns my partner on more than I realize, and he loves to see me show it off. 99

Attention deficit disorder

Now often diagnosed in childhood, ADHD is a common disease that affects a person's ability to stay focused, control his or her behavior, and interact in social settings. If left untreated or undiagnosed, the symptoms of ADHD can continue into adulthood, severely impacting your ability to form lasting, meaningful relationships.

Diagnosing ADHD

ADHD often goes undiagnosed in adults, particularly in adult women. This is because people tend to stereotype ADHD as a masculine disorder due to certain characteristics like hyperactivity (which is not often present in adults to begin with) and an inability to concentrate. However, more and more doctors are realizing that ADHD can affect anyone, regardless of gender, and that men and women might exhibit symptoms differently.

Sadly, women with undiagnosed ADHD can struggle with everything from depression to substance abuse to low self-esteem. If you struggle with this disease, you might find that it's hard to stay focused or finish tasks, which often leads to frustration and anxiety. You might also have difficulty keeping a conversation going or staying focused on the task at hand.

The truth about...

TREATING ADHD

While there is no cure for ADHD, there are many treatments that can help to decrease symptoms. In addition to medication, behavioral therapy can include relaxation techniques, exercise, and coping skills for times when you feel overwhelmed. Following certain routines and breaking your to-do list down into smaller tasks (e.g. "Put clothes in the washer" as opposed to "Do the laundry") can help make each goal easier to tackle. Working through negative thoughts and building self-esteem is also important, as many people with ADHD feel helpless or depressed because they aren't "normal" or "can't succeed."

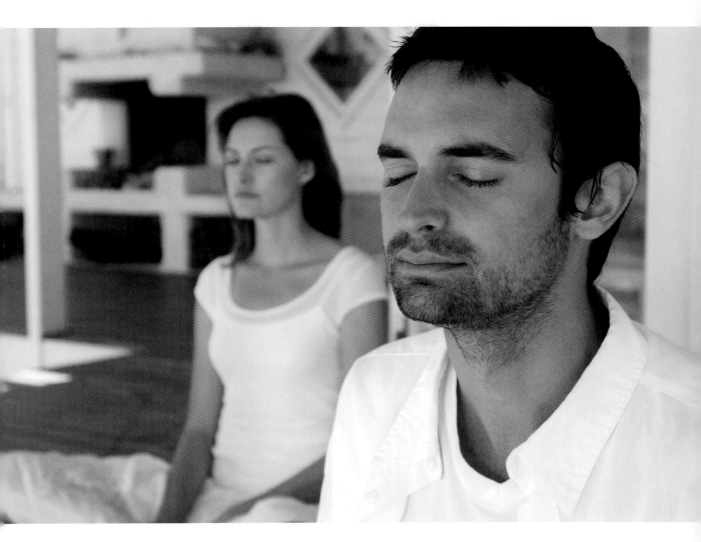

ADHD and relationships

Anything that disturbs your mental well-being can prevent you from finding and keeping the love you want. When ADHD is undiagnosed, you might find that your self-esteem suffers because you don't understand your scattered behavior and thoughts. You might feel out of control, frustrated, overwhelmed, or unable to commit in a relationship.

I find in my practice that women living with ADHD are under a great deal of stress. Sexually speaking, women with ADHD often struggle to reach orgasm because their minds are constantly multitasking, and they are unable to stay fully present in sexual scenarios. Until diagnosis and management of symptoms are achieved, it can be very hard to develop and maintain happy relationships.

Seeking therapy

Therapy is not just for people going through a difficult time or struggling with a diagnosed mental disorder. Even happy, secure people can benefit from having a safe place to express their emotions and delve into their inner selves. Committing to a mental health program is often the most positive choice a person can make, especially because therapy can be foundational in finding and keeping a good relationship. When you are in a healthy place emotionally, you are able to attract and bond with someone who is equally stable, confident, and happy.

Therapy techniques

Therapy has changed a great deal in recent years. If you have never been to therapy, you might picture it to be a Freudian experience, couch and all. Some therapy offices do have a couch, but that doesn't mean that you have to spend the time having your dreams interpreted, or even that you have to lie down. In reality, there are many types of therapy, as well as many types of therapists, and different types work best for different people and conditions.

Talk therapy, or "insight-oriented" therapy, is the most well-known type of therapy and originally derived from Sigmund Freud's therapy practice, although today most clinicians have departed greatly from his style. In talk therapy, the therapist asks questions and listens without judgment to a person's emotional situation. He or she can help you identify behaviors that are disruptive to your life, and help you examine the possible roots of those behaviors. The goal in talk therapy is to gain insight into the things that are keeping you from having the life you want, and provide the necessary healing in order to move beyond them.

Cognitive behavioral therapy differs from talk therapy in that sessions tend to focus more on the present than the past, helping you focus on new ways to cope with current stressors. You will learn how to recognize triggers or thoughts that lead you to undesired feelings or behaviors, and will also learn how to reshape your ways of thinking and acting in order to achieve a more positive outcome.

Group therapy is as simple as it sounds. This type of therapy helps individuals learn coping mechanisms and lessons from other people in similar situations. Examples include 12-step meetings, such as Overeaters Anonymous and Alcoholics Anonymous.

Behavioral therapy can help you become empowered in situations that would normally cause you to feel out of control or helpless. A behavioral therapist focuses on concrete behaviors and actions that you can practice to build the life and relationships that you want. This might involve learning social skills to help overcome specific fears or discovering concentration techniques to help you focus in the present more easily.

Drug therapy refers to the new mental health medications, which are used to treat everything from depression to obsessive-compulsive disorder to anxiety to sleep disturbances. Although these drugs can be very useful, they should typically be accompanied by another mode of therapy. Simply medicating a problem away is not a good solution, although it can be part of a good solution. This is why it's so important to talk to a psychiatrist rather than a medical practitioner—although your medical practitioner can be a useful starting point in helping you to find a therapist who is right for you.

New types of therapy

There are many other types of therapy, and more models are being established every year. Recently, types of creative therapy have become increasingly popular. Drama therapy, music therapy, writing therapy, art therapy, and wilderness therapy are just a handful of the creative, nonthreatening approaches that are helping people to improve their lives and mental well-being. You can experiment with different types of therapy to find what works best for you, or even combine different models in order to create your own customized program. You can also combine couples' therapy with individual therapy, or seek therapy as an individual but occasionally bring in your partner in order to seek help with conflict resolution.

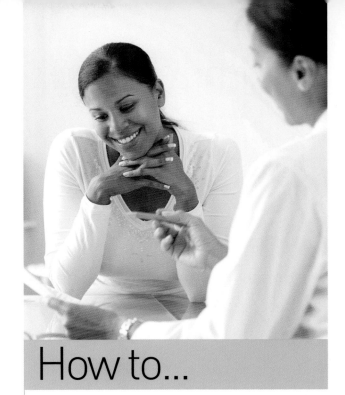

How to...

FIND THE RIGHT THERAPIST

Your relationship with your therapist is very personal, and can be a powerful part of the healing process that allows you to get the life you want and enter into relationships successfully. Spend some time looking for the right person. The steps below can help.

1 Identify your needs, and what type of therapy you are interested in. Then, think about what type of person would make you feel comfortable. Do you want a man or a woman? Someone your age or someone older who you might more easily view as a mentor? These specifics will help you search.

2 Ask friends and family members who have been through therapy to recommend people. Compile a list of names of people who might meet your needs.

3 Ask for recommendations from your medical practitioner, too.

4 Try several therapists until you find one who makes you feel comfortable and relaxed.

Maximizing your upper limits

Have you ever spent your whole week eagerly looking forward to Friday night? Then when Friday finally arrives and you get to spend much-needed R&R time with your partner, all you can do is argue? On the surface, it might seem like you are fighting about which restaurant has the best sushi or which movie to see, but the truth is, you are probably being held back by your own upper limits.

Your brain set

Stop and think about a moment when you felt full of joy, peace, and fulfillment. That place is where you are at your body's essence, and it is different for every person, with one important similarity—we would all like to stay in that place all of the time!

Unfortunately, we don't stay there all the time, and this is where the idea of upper limits comes in. The concept is pretty simple. Each of us has what experts now call a "brain set." Our brain set determines how much joy we can experience before our nervous systems and our minds start to become stressed. Once the upper limits of our brain set are reached, we feel out of our element and become nervous or uncomfortable, which causes us to unconsciously act or think in a way that brings us back down below our individual threshold. So, returning to our Friday night example, when you finally get home and are feeling excited about the evening ahead, you might begin to hit that threshold and thus feel compelled to retreat to a lower level of happiness. For example, you might start an argument with your partner, or begin dwelling on other worries. You may even start to look at a larger picture, wondering if it's right to be happy when there is so much suffering in the world.

Clearly, if you are bringing yourself (and perhaps your partner) down every time you start to experience joy, the quality of your relationship will be compromised. You will be more likely to unconsciously sabotage a special date, a vacation you've been looking forward to, or even an amazing sexual experience.

Our brain set is believed to be a result of our genes, our mental health, and how we were raised (our family's brain set). A person who suffers from anxiety or depression will have a lower brain set, or happiness threshold, than someone who doesn't suffer from these disorders. If you grew up in a family where one or both of your caregivers were

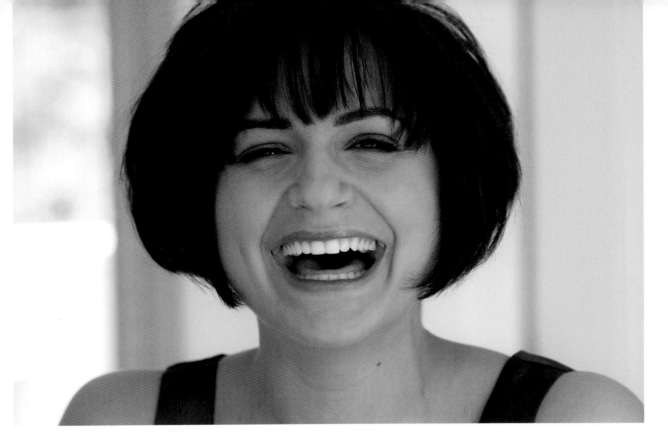

constantly worried or depressed, or didn't allow for great expressions of joy, your brain set may be lower. If you grew up in a family that was playful and silly, and allowed for open and deep experiences of joy and even sorrow, your brain set might be higher.

Patterns of happiness

There are three primary patterns of happiness, which can help us understand the way our individual brain set works. These are illustrated in the line graphs on the following page.

The happiness jumper experiences brief periods of extreme joy, then lapses into thought patterns that send his or her happiness levels plummeting. This type of person might be on top of the world one day and then struggle to get out of bed the next. During brief "up" periods, he or she may experience great sex and great love, but these moments always give way to times of sadness on the downward slope.

The happiness neutralizer never experiences great joy, intense passion, or great sorrow, but instead chooses to stay neutral in the middle. He or she never truly experiences amazing, soulful sex or intense joy, but also never experiences severe depression.

The happiness builder is the type of personality that we want to work toward. The happiness builder slowly but continually increases his or her happiness threshold, believing that our bodies, our minds, and our nervous systems need time to adjust to each new level of joy. This type of lifestyle avoids the yo-yo existence of the happiness jumper and experiences much deeper joy than the happiness neutralizer. As happiness builders slowly increase their capacity for joy, they also increase their capacity for sexual intensity, playfulness, experimentation, adventure, and connection in their relationships. Many experts who study brain sets believe that there is no limit to the amount of joy that we can experience in our lives.

Happiness patterns

Where do you fall on the graphs below? Are you a happiness jumper, constantly experiencing extreme highs and lows? Are you a happiness neutralizer, playing it safe with mediocre levels of joy? Or are you a happiness builder who is able to progress to deeper levels of joy over time? This last type of happiness growth is what we all want to achieve.

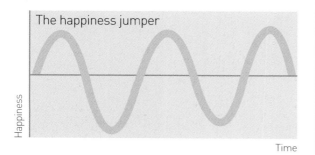

The happiness jumper

Happiness

Time

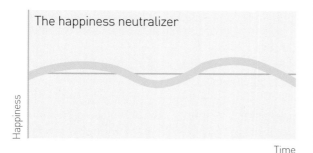

The happiness neutralizer

Happiness

Time

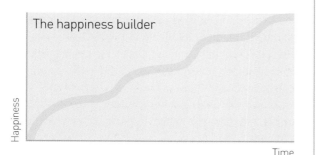

The happiness builder

Happiness

Time

Changing your brain set

The good news is that you can actually change your brain set in order to increase your upper limits. Medication is one way to do this. If you are depressed or anxious, you can begin taking antidepressants or other medications recommended by your doctor. These can help you relax, let go of worries, and feel more comfortable living in the present.

Another way to change your brain set is to notice when you are experiencing an upper limit and practice slowly expanding your happiness threshold. This will help you become a happiness builder. First, simply notice the fact that you are reaching your upper limits. Don't become angry or frustrated with yourself. Instead, try to consciously work on letting go of these limits and allowing yourself to move beyond them. To do this, work backward and examine what thoughts have led to your emotional state. Are you concerned that you will get stuck in traffic on your way home from work? Are you worried the babysitter will call and cancel again? Allow yourself to see that even if these situations occur, your evening need not be ruined. When you accept that you cannot control these circumstances, but can control your thoughts and actions, you can free yourself from the stress of trying to create the "perfect" life.

The truth is that nothing is every going to be perfect. You are never going to have a perfect vacation or a perfect weekend. You might lose your wallet, it might rain every day, or your kid might get a sore throat. Learning to take these challenges in stride is an important part of being a mature and happy adult.

Postponing pleasure

Another threat to becoming a happiness builder is the practice of "storing up" pleasure for the future, or, essentially, planning to be happy at some future date. People who do this are basically setting themselves up for disaster. While it's natural to look forward to a vacation or a weekend activity with your partner, it's unhealthy to constantly feel the need to create a perfect experience. Friday night is, after all, just… Friday night. There is no reason to funnel all of your energy and excitement into one night a week. It is much better to seek joy in every activity than to place too much importance on a few moments.

Additionally, if postponing pleasure becomes a habit, it begins to feel much more natural than actually experiencing pleasure. This makes it doubly important to stop storing up happiness for some future date. You can connect with your loved ones and appreciate your life even if you aren't relaxing on a beach in Mexico. And, funnily enough, once you learn to do this, you will enjoy that beach vacation twice as much, because you will have finally learned to manage your upper limits.

Living in the now

One way to put yourself in a place that allows joyfulness at every moment of the day is to practice staying in the moment, or "living in the now," as some call it. The concept of living in the now is quite simple, but also quite revolutionary. When you live in the now, you make a conscious choice to only concern yourself with the present. This means that there is no obsessing about what went wrong yesterday or what may go wrong tomorrow or next year.

The good news is that it's not as hard as it sounds. You can stay in the present by simply bringing awareness and consciousness to your being every time you realize you aren't living in the now. Once you start practicing this, you might be surprised at how much time you waste thinking about the embarrassing thing you said two years ago, or worrying over your toddler's college fund, or stressing about the impression you made at your partner's holiday party. All of these fears hold you back from embracing true happiness. The only time that is promised to you is the present, and enjoying that time is the best way to feel truly happy (see Resources, page 251, for tools that can help you learn more about this life-changing technique).

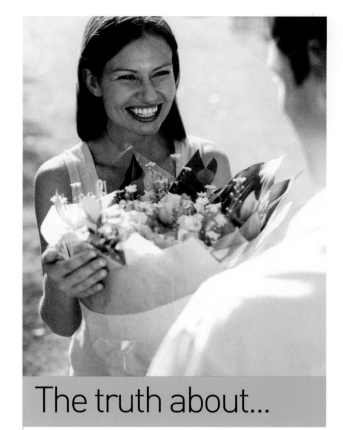

The truth about...

LIMITING HAPPINESS

It's your anniversary. You have been secretly planning for this day, buying your partner a sweet card, purchasing sexy lingerie, and even getting your hair and nails done. Then, the day rolls around and your partner sends you flowers at work. He takes you out for a nice dinner. But the whole time you can't help thinking, "This is it?" You want fireworks and over-the-top gestures so much that you don't realize that happiness is right in front of you.

We all build up expectations in our heads that can never be fully met. When you notice this, simply relax, notice the little pleasures that surround you, and make a choice to let your happiness flow freely.

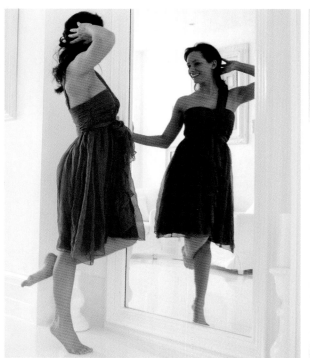
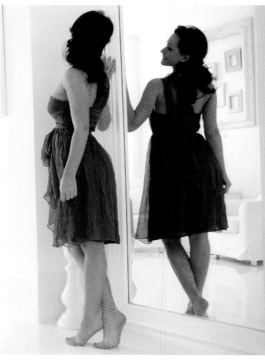

Chapter 4

Reconnecting with your body

Your body is one of your most precious gifts, and how you take care of it truly impacts your happiness and quality of life. Eating healthily and exercising regularly can help you stay present in your relationship, enjoy your daily routine, and promote a joy-filled outlook in every area of your life. Just as important, it can give you the confidence to fully enjoy an adventurous, intimate sex life.

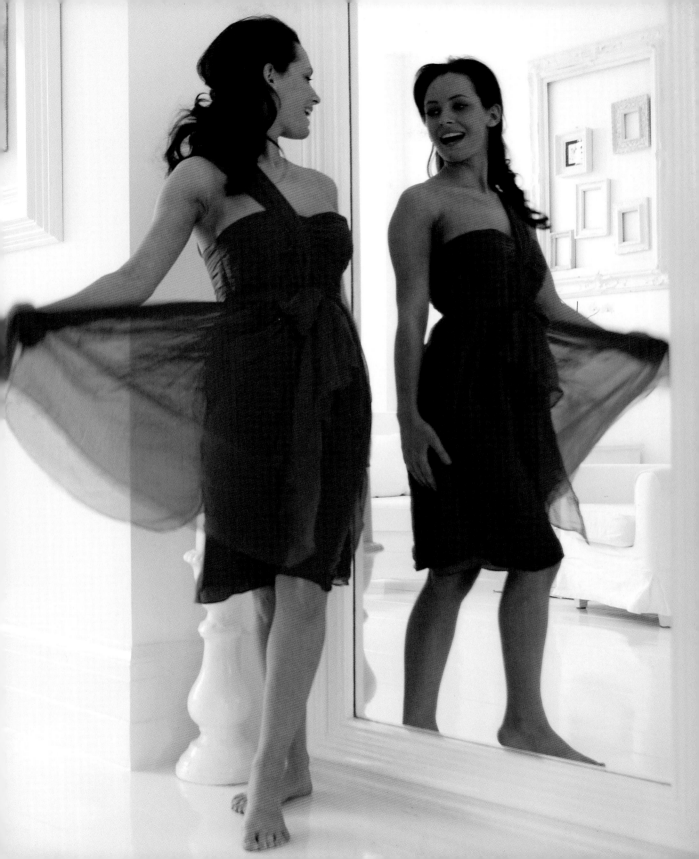

A healthy body is an important part of a healthy mindset and relationship.

Regardless of your age or physical fitness, the food you eat and the way you treat your body will determine everything from your self-esteem to your body's functioning to your sexual success. And yet, most of us treat our bodies thoughtlessly or even disdainfully, neglecting to spend the time to take care of our most important belonging.

This chapter will help you adjust the way you think about and treat your body, so that you can enter or move forward in a relationship with confidence. As a starting point, reflect on your body image by taking the quiz below, considering your response to each question carefully and honestly.

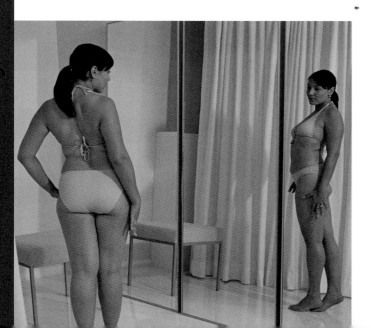

1 YOUR FRIEND CALLS YOU AND ASKS YOU TO COME to an exclusive restaurant opening with her. Your first thought is:

Ⓐ "I can't wait to get dressed up and enjoy a night on the town!"

Ⓑ "Is she crazy? I don't have a dress that fits and I am not going to go looking like a fatso. She'll have to find a skinnier friend."

Ⓒ "There is no way I am going to blow my diet just for one night of fun."

2 IN JUST A FEW WEEKS, YOU AND YOUR HUSBAND are headed to Florida to enjoy some time on the beach without the kids. It's the first vacation you've taken alone together in two years. You are:

Ⓐ Excited about all the romance and sex! It's been forever since it was just the two of you enjoying each other's company as lovers instead of parents.

Ⓑ In the middle of a grueling cleanse. You have to lose at least 10 pounds in the next two weeks or you won't be caught dead in a swimsuit.

Ⓒ Frantically calling the resort to grill their staff for details about the gym and the low-carb diet plan offered at the restaurant.

3 YOU DECIDE TO ATTEMPT A 5K FOR A CHARITABLE CAUSE and to lose some weight. By the third week of training, you are:

Ⓐ Tired and a little sore, but still showing up to practice every afternoon. You only wish you could say the same for your friend who signed up with you and then bailed after week one.

B Completely frustrated and close to giving up. You have been working hard and starving yourself on limited calories, but you still don't have the perfect body you were dreaming of.

C Bragging about your latest track time to anyone who will listen and trying to pressure your partner to join in and "lose some of that gut."

4 IT'S FRIDAY, AND YOU'VE HAD A LONG, HARD WEEK.
You decide to:

A Go to yoga class as planned, and then come home and enjoy a helping of fettuccine alfredo, a healthy salad, and a glass of wine.

B Forget your diet, eat an entire pizza, and drink several glasses of wine.

C Flake on plans with your sister because you want to spend extra time on the treadmill at the gym.

5 IT'S YOUR FIFTEENTH WEDDING ANNIVERSARY,
and you decide you want to buy some special lingerie to commemorate the occasion. At the store, you:

A Grab a bunch of sexy stuff to try on and hit the fitting room, excited about finding the perfect outfit for the night.

B Walk through the store dejected, deciding that you won't be caught dead in any of their lingerie with your cellulite and "thunder thighs."

C Splurge on at least five different things, and make a mental note not to eat too much at dinner so you don't look bloated in your new sexy garb.

6 YOU AND YOUR PARTNER MAKE A NEW YEAR'S PACT TO BECOME HEALTHIER.
To accomplish this goal, you:

A Begin getting up 30 minutes earlier so you can go for a run before work, and start actually making meals from your low-carb cookbooks.

B Pin pictures of models up around your bathroom mirror to remind you both how far you have to go to reach your desired weights.

C Create a strict 1,200-calorie diet plan for you and your partner, and begin working out twice a day.

7 YOUR FIRST BABY WAS BORN SIX MONTHS AGO.
You love being a mother, but miss your pre-baby figure. To get in shape, you:

A Cut back on your chocolate intake and recommit to your unused gym membership by signing up for Pilates classes three mornings a week.

B Make the switch to two small meals a day, but still succumb to late-night ice cream binges.

C Restructure your entire schedule to accommodate lengthy sessions with your new trainer.

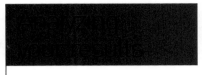

A-type answers indicate that you have a healthy attitude toward fitness, nutrition, and your body. You understand the importance of exercise and a balanced diet, but you also allow yourself to enjoy special occasions and feel good about yourself regardless of your weight.

B-type answers may mean that you are stuck in a rut of negative body image. You often skip meals and try punishing diets in an attempt to lose weight quickly, but all that deprivation causes you to ricochet into over-indulging. You don't feel comfortable in your own body, and it affects your self-esteem and even your sex life.

C-type answers suggest that you are committed to a healthy lifestyle, but you might be overdoing it. You are obsessed with calorie counting and weight loss. Remember, it's important to find balance—so keep hitting the gym, but don't overdo it. If you feel like you can't let go of strict exercise or diet requirements, or if you often experience negative feelings about your body, see page 70 for more on eating disorders.

❝The way you treat your body will determine everything from your self-esteem to your sexual success.**❞**

Redefining healthy living

Truly committing to living a healthy life is difficult, especially when you think that you should put other's food preferences above your own. Maybe your family begs you to order pizza and you give in, even though you were planning on preparing chicken and veggies. Or your best friend convinces you to overindulge in margaritas and fajitas after work. For most of us, situations like these are all too familiar. It's hard to stand up to the people closest to us when it comes to a healthy eating regime, especially when we are secretly dying for a slice of pizza (or two, or three)! But stay strong. The benefits of healthy living are huge, not just for your personal health but for your relationship and your sexuality.

Making healthy choices

Part of the problem is that we have a skewed idea about what healthy living means: We think that it is boring or time-consuming, or that it turns you into one of those people who only wants to talk about calories. Of course, this can happen, and some people are overly obsessed with health. But it doesn't have to. You don't have to become a gym rat who measures out the calories in apple slices. Instead, you can make small healthy choices throughout the day, whether it is to order a salad without creamy dressing, or to not drink soda, or to take the stairs instead of the elevator. Healthy choices add up over time, and even though you won't lose weight dramatically right away, you will eventually see a difference in how you look and feel.

So, this is the most important first step: You have to change the way that you think about healthy living. This is especially true when it comes to food. Often, people see healthy foods as a punishment and unhealthy foods as a tasty reward. In other words, salads, vegetables, and other healthy foods are just part of the masochistic journey to a flatter tummy, while foods like burgers and pizza are what really make you happy. Sure, certain foods taste good in the moment, but you likely know from firsthand experience that you feel better mentally and physically after a healthy meal than you do after splurging on a bunch of junk food.

Motivating change

Making this thought change is all about removing the mindset that healthy foods and exercise are negative. Think about it: What's negative about enjoying food created by Mother Nature herself, as opposed to food created in a factory? If you reflect on where your food is coming from, as opposed to simply eating whatever tastes good, you might find that the most tempting junk foods are actually quite

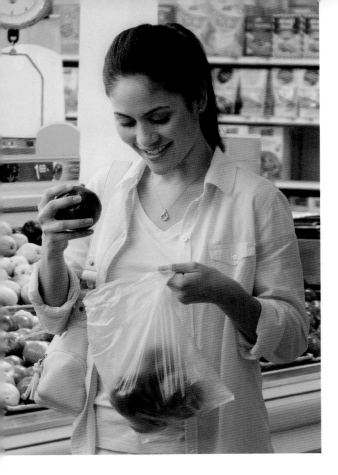

> **66** The more you think about what you are eating, the more likely you will be to eat consciously. **99**

Healthy living and your sex life

Your mind, body, and spirit are all connected. When you physically don't feel your best, it impacts your entire life in ways you might not even realize. You may not have the energy for sex, or you may get sick more easily. If you are overweight and self-conscious about your body, these ramifications might become even more extreme. You might avoid pool parties or the very idea of lingerie because you are embarrassed by your body. As a result, you might miss out on enjoyable times with friends or intimate moments with your partner. When you start to make choices out of fear or embarrassment, such as wanting to hide your body, your self-esteem is affected, and causes a ripple effect of negativity throughout your life.

So, exercising and eating healthily is not only about weight, but about supporting your immune system, your energy, and your overall sense of well-being, which in turn strengthens your relationships. If you hate the thought of restrictive diets or counting calories, don't worry. That's not what a healthy lifestyle is about. Instead, it's about committing to your health and happiness by eating real food and getting active a few times a week. These small changes are easy to incorporate into your life and yet they also have the ability to revolutionize your self-confidence and relationships.

horrifying. From chemicals to preservatives to hormones, most of the packaged foods that you find in the supermarket are more like a science experiment than a satisfying meal. Even the animals we eat aren't always being fed healthy foods—they are being pumped full of hormones and vaccines, and the vegetables we consume are often covered in pesticides. This doesn't mean that you have to be a strict organic vegan who only eats raw foods, but it does mean that you should value your body enough to stop and think about what you are putting into it. The more you think about what you are eating, the more likely you will be to eat as naturally and consciously as possible. And, once you start making these healthy choices, you will find that you start to crave nutritious foods. Even better, your new, healthy eating habits can be hugely motivating to friends and family members.

Nutrition

Healthy eating is a choice that we have to make every time we sit down to eat, whether we are hovering over our desk at work or enjoying a meal with our families. Making these choices isn't always easy, but embarking on a nutritious life will be one of the most rewarding journeys you will ever take. Of course, no one is perfect, and you will likely experience a few setbacks, but don't allow one day of unhealthy eating to derail your commitment to change. Tomorrow is another day to start again.

Organic eating

One of the easiest ways to motivate healthy nutrition choices is to notice and be thankful for the variety of fresh foods available, from seasonal fruits to fresh, organic vegetables to farm-fresh produce. Banish the idea that you are being punished or cheated if you aren't indulging in a burrito or satisfying a snack craving with a bag of cheesy chips. Instead, stick to eating things that your great grandmother would recognize as food (i.e. not something you can generally find at a drive-through window). This means opting for fresh, organic food wherever possible.

Watch out for preservatives and make it a point to stay away from simple carbohydrates and white flour. Many people have undiagnosed allergies to wheat and yeast, which can make them feel lethargic and may cause headaches and rashes. Even without allergies, you may feel bloated and fatigued if your diet is too carb-heavy, so limit your carbohydrate intake, and opt for whole grains whenever possible. To start, try switching to whole-wheat cereal. Or, try sweet potatoes instead of baked potatoes, and mashed cauliflower instead of mashed potatoes.

If you suspect you have a food allergy, start keeping a food diary and note when symptoms occur. Your doctor can then help you decipher if you have an allergy, and how best to treat it.

Nutrition and sexuality

Have you ever felt like you were having an "off" day physically, and were consequently less interested in sex? It wasn't just your emotions playing tricks on you—science shows that when we are not healthy, we are less interested in sex. In addition to draining your energy and health, high-fat, high-sugar, and high-carb foods can also negatively impact your sex drive and your sexual pleasure. Extra weight makes you lethargic, weak, and sluggish—all things that hurt you when you are chasing after the big "O."

Eating consciously

Most of us will try anything when it comes to weight loss, whether it is the grapefruit diet, the Master Cleanse, or a low-carb plan. Mealtime becomes an exercise in miserable self-restraint, often made worse by the fact that the people around us are eating something temptingly high in calories. Luckily, there is a better way than all these over-hyped diet plans. If you are looking to lose weight or commit to a healthy lifestyle, my number one tip is to start eating consciously. Bring awareness and enjoyment back to mealtime, and feed your body real, nutritious food. You will feel better and look better as a result! The ideas below will get you started.

Make cooking fun. People often think of cooking as a chore, but the truth is, it can be one of the best parts of your day. There are many healthy and delicious meals that can be prepared in 30 minutes or less. Enlist your kids to help set the table or wash the vegetables, while you take control of the chopping and sautéing. When you actually prepare real food, you will feel more involved and satiated by what you eat—and it sure beats poking a few holes in a Lean Cuisine and sticking it in the microwave.

Start a new tradition in your family. We have all heard the studies that say that family dinners are beneficial for our children's well-being, but they can also be beneficial for parents. Dinnertime is your time to enjoy your family and focus on the people who matter the most. Make a family commitment to turn off the television and ignore any calls or emails for at least 30 minutes during dinnertime. The bonus: When you focus on the meal at hand, rather than shoveling in bites during *American Idol*, you will pay more attention to tasting and enjoying your food, which means you will eat less and feel more satisfied.

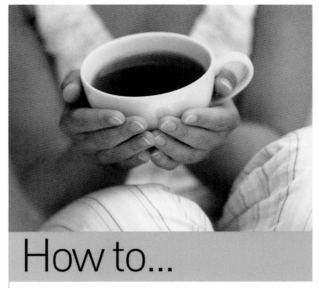

How to...

START YOUR HEALTHY LIFESTYLE

Remember that eating healthily isn't just about cutting back on empty calories. Many foods, including caffeine and refined sugar, negatively impact the functioning of the body. You will have more energy, and your sweet-tooth cravings will naturally decrease as you limit your sugar indulgence. Try the tips below to get started.

1 Cut back on your coffee and soda intake, one cup at a time. Gradually swap out your coffee for green tea and your soda for water or fresh juice.

2 Commit to cutting out refined sugar for one week (honey and agave nectar are okay). At the end of the week, notice how much more energy you have and how much better you feel.

3 Find a farmer's market near you. Shopping for fresh, farm-to-table produce is both fun and inexpensive. Make it a Saturday morning ritual.

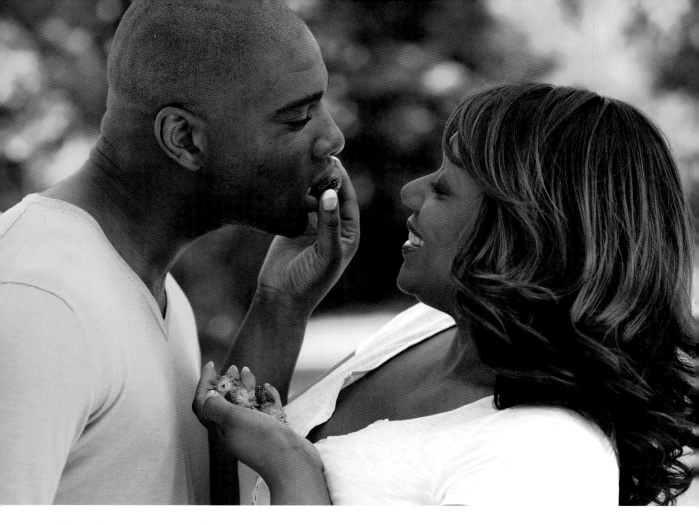

Planning your meals

Planning ahead is one of the best ways to monitor what you eat—and, in fact, how you eat is almost as important as what you eat. Small meals throughout the day will keep you satisfied and will help you maintain a healthy metabolism. It will also protect you from filling up on calories whenever hunger strikes, and will give you more energy throughout the day.

It is epecially important to plan your meals at home if you have young kids who tend to take up a lot of your attention during dinnertime. In fact, you might consider serving the kids first, and then having a "grown-up" dinner with your partner later. This will allow you to taste your food and enjoy it, rather than focusing solely on trying to keep order at the table.

It might seem harder to plan your meals when you are eating out, but you can actually follow the same rules you do at home: Really think about what you're putting in your body, and don't overindulge. Remember that diners tend to eat excess calories when dining out. Avoid the bread basket and try to eat only half of your entrée, then stop eating when you are full, rather than polishing off your entire plate. One of the nicest things about going out with your partner is that it can inject a little romance into your normal routine. However, stuffing yourself with calories is one sure-fire way to put a damper on romance. If you truly believe that you are what you eat, than a greasy pizza is hardly going to make you feel sexy. The lighter the meal, the lighter you feel, and the more energy you have for intimacy.

Sensual eating

Your eating rituals can make all the difference in your mealtime experience. Don't just zone out in front of the television or rush through your meal without thinking. Instead, make sensual eating a practice. Use all of your senses when you eat. For example, if you are eating an orange, notice how you can feel the texture of the skin as you peel it; you can smell the citrus scent; you can see its deep, rich color; and you can taste the juices as you eat it, one piece at a time. Practicing this type of food appreciation will not only help you stay conscious about what you are eating, it will also help you get more closely in touch with your sensual side. To reap the benefits of sensual eating even more, encourage your partner to join you—then watch as this conscious approach to eating makes your relationship naturally steamier.

Cook together. Cooking can be a very sensual experience. Don an apron, open a bottle of wine, and listen to some music while you and your partner make dinner together. Not only will it give you a chance to talk and bond, but feeling, tasting, and smelling food will awaken your sensuality. Experiment with new recipes and have fun with food. Even the most inexperienced chefs can make low-fat pasta or a delectable seafood entrée.

Practice sensual eating. One of the best ways to do this as a couple is to incorporate all of your senses into intimacy. Try playing with edible body paint, feeding each other, or licking food off each other. Use simple, sensual, classic foods, such as fruit, chocolate, or whipped cream.

Indulge in a tasting adventure. Plan a tasting date for just the two of you or for a group of friends. Pair foods with regional wines, or step a bit off the beaten path and try a honey, olive oil, or chocolate tasting. Smell, sample, and savor the differences you taste.

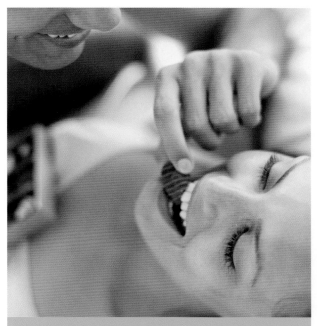

The truth about...

NATURAL APHRODISIACS

Although there is no clinical study that proves the existence of aphrodisiacs, foods like chocolate have been shown to influence pleasure areas of the brain, so indulging in a piece of dark chocolate may help you to relax and feel more sensual. Need more convincing? A study completed by Italian researcher Dr. Andrea Salonia demonstrated a link between satisfying sex and chocolate.

Many people also report feeling more amorous after a glass of wine, but that's most likely because their inhibitions are down. Beware of overindulging when it comes to alcohol! Too much will kill your libido and diminish sensation. For a healthier way to add some spice, foods such as jalapenos help speed up metabolism and might get your heart racing for more spicy activities in the bedroom.

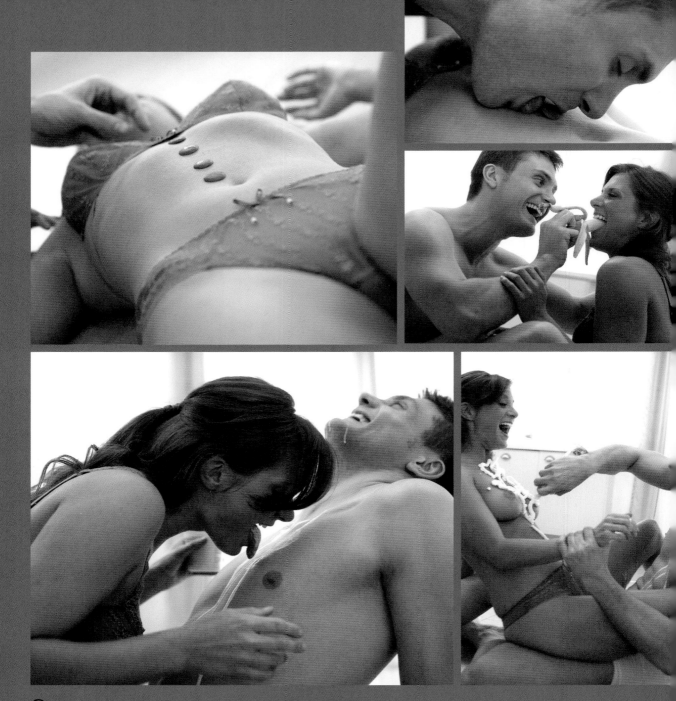

Sweet treat

One trick that's guaranteed to spice up the way you think about food is to plan an erotic bedroom picnic. Start with sensual classics like chocolate, whipped cream, and strawberries—and, of course, you, your partner, and some mouthwatering lingerie. Then, get as playful and creative as you dare. Taste, touch, and tempt your way through an evening of pure, decadent fantasy.

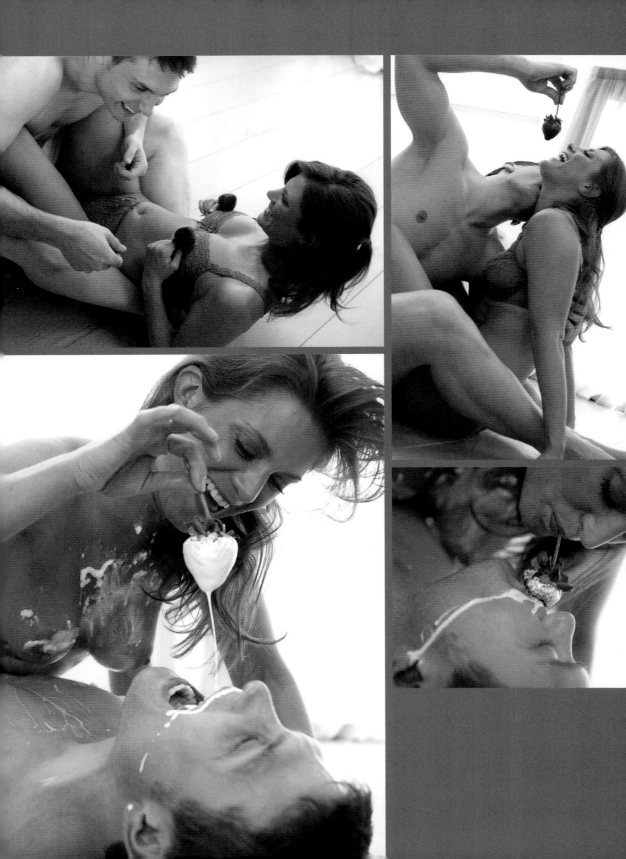

Exercise

Exercise is not something that most of us enjoy. After all, who wants to leave the office at the end of a long day and go sweat in the gym? It's much easier to just go home and get comfortable on the couch. Yet, physically and emotionally, our bodies crave exercise. We aren't meant to be sedentary. Our bodies are designed to move, whether that movement is swimming, dancing, running, boxing, walking, or any of dozens of other ways to stay active.

Personalizing your fitness

This is the good news: Exercise is personal. You can tailor it to fit your interests, your schedule, and your natural abilities. You can squeeze exercise in at times that work best for you, such as during your lunch hour or before the kids wake up in the morning. You can take a dance class with your best friend, start a jogging club with other moms in your neighborhood, or even try a new activity like rock climbing or tennis. Remember that there are many ways to stay active and healthy that don't involve a treadmill. Consider the ideas below as you get started creating a personal fitness plan.

Find little ways to work exercise into your day, whether it's taking the stairs instead of the elevator, parking on the far side of the parking lot, or biking to work when it's nice outside.

Get active with your kids during the evenings by playing with them in the backyard, going to the park, or even playing a video fitness game, such as Wii.

Carry a pedometer and make it your goal to walk 8,000–10,000 steps a day. (The average person walks 5,000–7,000 steps a day.)

Becoming motivated

The next time you find yourself dreading the gym or opting not to exercise, think about what's preventing you from committing to yourself. Is it because you juggle a busy work and social schedule, and don't have time? Is it because you feel you should spend time with your kids instead? In reality, few priorities will yield more benefits than taking care of your physical health. Remember that your kids need a healthy parent who is committed to fitness—so if you can't find a babysitter, do something active with the kids. The more exercise becomes part of your regular routine, the easier it will be to maintain a fitness schedule without letting daily obstacles get in your way. In time, you may even find that you genuinely look forward to this part of your day.

This is important because our minds crave exercise as well. Physical activity releases feel-good endorphins and helps ease the buildup of stress. Additionally, when we commit to a healthy exercise program and stick to it, we feel strong, powerful, and proud of our achievements. Going home and sitting on the couch might feel good in the moment, but going to the gym feels good far into the future.

Thinking positively

One way to change your mental attitude toward fitness is to follow up every negative thought with a positive thought. Positivity is much more effective than negativity. You can only motivate

> 66 Our minds crave exercise, too: it releases feel-good endorphins and helps ease stress. 99

with negative energy for so long, which is why so many women burn out after a while. Your mind can only take so much self-hatred before it collapses and returns to its pizza-loving ways. This is why it's best to stop thoughts like: "I am so fat, I have to spend at least an hour at the gym tonight." Instead, motivate yourself with positive and hopeful plans,

Sweating off stress

Simply put, exercise is one of the very best ways to de-stress. Any type of physical activity releases nerve-calming endorphins in your brain, which can work wonders on your mood and help you relax. Here are a few of the ways that working out can calm you down.

Stress relief

- **As an outlet for negativity.** Run, dance, or stretch out those feelings of frustration, anger, and even sadness. When you renew and strengthen your body, your mind can't help but feel renewed as well.
- **As a social tool.** Joining a gym or a sports team is a great way to meet new people, which can help you feel connected and involved in your community.
- **As a sleep enhancer.** Physical exercise uses up excess stores of adrenalin, which can calm you down and help you sleep at night.
- **As a worry reducer.** When you exercise, you rest the nerve cells in your brain that worry, giving them time to renew so they can continue functioning properly. Exercise also gives you an immediate goal to focus on, allowing your mind to take a break from other goals that may be causing stress.

such as: "If I keep going to the gym, I am going to be so confident in my bikini." Or, instead of thinking about how working out will change your weight, think of how it will change your mood. You aren't just selling yourself false motivation. In fact, it is probably hard to think of a time when you have regretted exercising. This is a real clue that no matter how much you might dread the gym at times, exercising is truly the best thing for your health. All you have to do is listen to what your body's telling you.

In the end, it's not about being a size two, or even about weight loss at all. In fact, I often suggest that women who want to lose 15 pounds or less ignore the scale completely—even throw it out! Focus on how your body feels, how your clothes fit, how strong you are, and how your endurance has increased. Then, celebrate your gym victories and allow yourself to enjoy your favorite foods once in a while. In fitness as in life, it's all about balance.

The truth about...
EXERCISE IN HIGH HEELS

A study in Italy recently found that women who wear heels from time to time have better pelvic floor strength than women who don't. This is thought to be because the way you balance your body when you walk in stilettos causes you to tighten your transverse abdominal muscles—although don't forget wearing heels too often can be bad for your back.

So the next time you are walking in those sexy stilettos, think about tightening your abs and pelvic floor as you move. You'll feel more stable, your posture will be better, and your stomach will look flatter. Not to mention that you'll be getting a workout just by moving from Point A to Point B— a pretty good way to multi-task, if you ask me!

Sexy exercise

One of the most fun ways to add spice to your fitness routine is to add some sex-inspired movement. You can do this by strengthening your pelvic floor. The pelvic floor supports your internal organs including your bladder, uterus, and vagina. Improved pelvic floor strength can mean better and longer orgasms, and increased control over your sexual response.

One way to strengthen this part of your body is to exercise your transverse abdominal muscles, which are the lower ab muscles that surround the torso (also where many women tend to carry extra weight). Think of your abdominal muscles as a built-in corset, with two plates just below your belly and above your mons pubis. As you tighten and squeeze those muscles together, those plates slide over each other, knitting the corset together more tightly. These muscles hold your body upright, correct your posture, and support your spine and torso, so when you pull them together, you can feel your body immediately respond.

Any kind of exercise that works your core will help with pelvic floor strength. You can try golf, pilates, yoga, dance, or one of the simple at-home exercises below. Just be sure to consult your doctor before beginning a new fitness program.

The plank. Start with your elbows on the ground and your shoulders above your elbows. Then, extend your legs so that they are in a traditional pushup position. Contract your abs and hold your stomach in (don't arch your back). Hold this position for as long as you can, taking deep breaths and making sure to hold your core firm and tight.

Leg raises. Lie on your back with your arms by your sides. Contract your abs and breath in, raising your legs so they are at a 90-degree angle. Keep your lower back on the ground as you slowly lower your legs. You can perform this exercise with straight or bent legs, or raise one leg at a time instead of both.

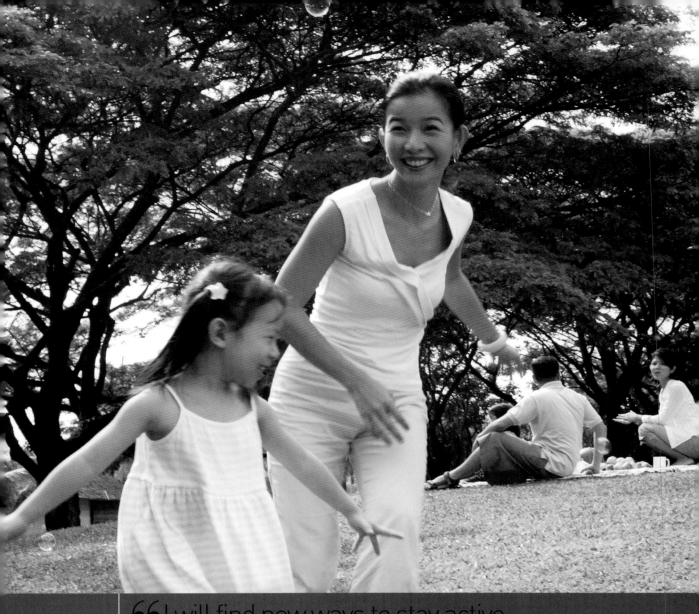

**"I will find new ways to stay active
and healthy, to enhance my lifestyle."**

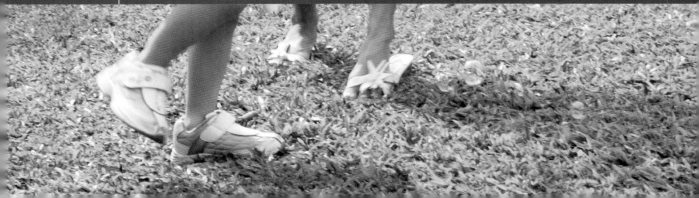

Self-stimulation

It's not often talked about, but knowing how to self-stimulate is a core part of being in touch with your body and your sexuality. In fact, for many women it is the foundation that allows them to lead happy, healthy, orgasmic lives with their partners. When you learn how to touch and pleasure your body, you awaken and enhance your sexual response. Even more important, you get reacquainted with yourself as a sexy and sexual being.

Why self-stimulate?

All too often, women (and men, for that matter) think that sex doesn't require any work. In part, this goes back once again to the way that movies and television have shaped our culture. We think that sex with the right person is always earth-shatteringly orgasmic. Let me remind you that that's simply not the case. Don't make the mistake of thinking that if you are with the right guy, if he knew how to touch the right button, then your sexual response would blossom and you'd experience real pleasure effortlessly.

The simple truth is that unless you figure it out for yourself, no one else will be able to bring you to that pleasurable place. And, unless you speak up about what works for you in the bedroom, your partner won't know. A woman who is fully satisfied and in control of her sex life not only knows her own body and how to stimulate it, she's able to communicate those needs to her partner (we'll get to that in just a couple of chapters). Self-stimulation is a great way for you to get to know your body and your sexual response, and it can also teach you to relax and enjoy pleasure without feeling self-conscious.

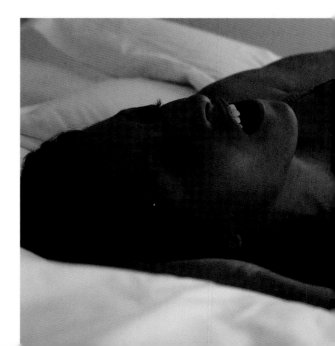

Getting started

If you have never tried self-stimulating before, or if you haven't been able to reach orgasm on your own, you might feel a little uncomfortable at the thought of a party for one. To start, try to set a calm, sensual mood that will help you relax. Put on some sexy music and perhaps even some of your favorite lingerie, and lock the door. If you want, wait for a time when no one is home, so you are absolutely sure there will be no distractions.

You can now explore your body to your heart's content. Begin by touching your clitoris, the center of female sexual pleasure. It is located at the top of your vulva, inside your labia, and is around the size of a small pea. As you become aroused, it will become larger and stiffer. Experiment with different strokes and pressures to see which feel best to you.

Next, try to locate your G-spot, another female hotspot. Your G-spot is located inside of your vagina, on your belly button side. It is about one-third of the way in, and you can locate it by making a come hither motion with your index finger. It feels spongy, much like the tip of your nose.

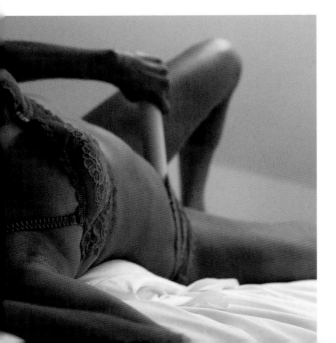

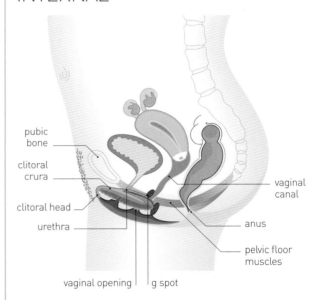

Female anatomy

INTERNAL

- pubic bone
- clitoral crura
- clitoral head
- urethra
- vaginal opening
- g spot
- vaginal canal
- anus
- pelvic floor muscles

EXTERNAL

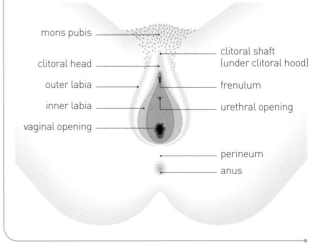

- mons pubis
- clitoral head
- outer labia
- inner labia
- vaginal opening
- clitoral shaft (under clitoral hood)
- frenulum
- urethral opening
- perineum
- anus

Dealing with long-term illness

Physical health and sexual health go hand in hand. When your physical health is lacking, your sexual health will be impacted. Yet even if you are committed to caring for your body, you might still have certain limitations in the bedroom. Such is the case for the millions of people who have long-term physical challenges, including mobility disorders, diabetes, cancer, or one of many other physically altering diseases. These require special treatment and consideration, but you can overcome them to have a healthy, happy sex life.

Mobility disorders

Mobility impairments include a wide range of disabilities some of which are temporary and some of which are permanent. They can be mild, or they can impact a person's entire life. Today, 25 million people suffer from mobility impairments, including paralysis, nerve damage, muscle weakness, stiff joints, or lack of balance or coordination.

Creativity can help your sexuality thrive despite mobility challenges. A good way to help get your sex life back on track is to look into sexual aids that are designed for your particular mobility challenge, whether you suffer from reduced mobility, nerve impairment, or even bowel or bladder concerns. For those who have reduced mobility, look for sex aids that come with a remote control or a long extension, which can help you give or receive sexual pleasure without unnecessary strain. For those with nerve impairment, powerful vibrators and pultrasonic vibrators can help deliver the stimulation you need for arousal and orgasm. For more about these and other sex aids, see pages 166–167.

Perhaps the best sexual aid for those with mobility issues is a good set of pillows. You can use them to support you to reduce joint strain, and to try different positions and angles. If you want to take it to the next level, look for furniture designed with sex in mind, like the Liberator. Pieces like this can be invaluable for minimizing joint strain and increasing sensation and stimulation. They can also offer quite a bit of erotic excitement: more advanced models include furniture equipped with submission and domination cuffs and waterproof material. There is truly something for people of every age, interest, and mobility level.

In addition, finding a comfortable and safe position to have sex is crucial, especially if you have back or knee issues. If your partner has a bad back, he might find that a seated position in which you are straddling

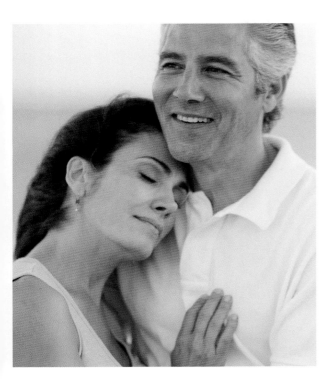

them!), because of the way the brain processes orgasms. For instance, even if you have no sensation from the waist down, you can learn to have an orgasm from having your ears kissed and stimulated. This is because when one sense is dulled, the other areas often take on greater sensation. In addition, research has found that Viagra can potentially be helpful in promoting arousal and orgasm in women with spinal cord injuries, and cervical stimulation can also help to improve your chances of reaching orgasm. The bottom line is that your sexuality is much more complex than meets the eye—so as long as there is a will, there is probably a way.

Fibromyalgia

Around two percent of Americans suffer from fibromyalgia, and women are more likely to be diagnosed with this disorder than men. Fibromyalgia causes widespread pain throughout the body, on both the right and left side, and above and below the waist. Although we do not know what causes fibromyalgia, it seems to often strike following a physical or emotional trauma, and to run in families, which suggests genetic predisposition. Fibromyalgia is also strongly connected with sleep disturbances, including sleep apnea, and many people with fibromyalgia find that they can sleep for hours without feeling rested or relaxed. Some doctors believe that this is because people with fibromyalgia never enter into a deep, restful sleep.

Your doctor may be able to suggest certain home remedies that can help decrease your pain and increase your sexual enjoyment. For example, taking a warm bath prior to sex can help alleviate muscle tenderness and swelling. Or, if the pain means that traditional sexual intercourse no longer works for you, remember that different sexual positions, mutual masturbation, and oral sex can

him is most comfortable. You can also try lying side by side or, if you are the one with joint issues, ask him to be on top. Find what is most comfortable for you and accessorize with sex aids if your desired position doesn't allow for the stimulation you need.

Spinal cord injury

Spinal cord injuries affect nearly 250,000 Americans. People with these injuries often find that their sexual function and response is affected, yet many of them are able to continue enjoying their sex life with a little bit of education and a commitment to communicating with a partner.

Ultimately, there are many ways to explore your sexuality, even if they are nontraditional. In fact, research has shown that many women with spinal cord injuries can still have climaxes (and plenty of

> **66** With a commitment to open communication, you can embrace your sexuality regardless of disability. **99**

still be enjoyable and are all excellent ways of maintaining intimacy. In addition, the more connected you are to your partner, the less stress you will experience and the more you will enjoy sex.

Decreasing stress is also crucial in treating fibromyalgia. When possible, light exercise is a good way to release endorphins and decrease stress, as are meditation and breathing exercises. Other forms of therapy such as music, reading, and painting can all help treat stress. It is also important to embrace the fact that your sex life might have to change as a result of fibromyalgia.

Cancer

As all-consuming as cancer often is, there is no reason why cancer patients can't enjoy a fulfilling sex life. In fact, committing to your sexuality can help improve your emotional health and decrease stress and depression, which can greatly improve your physical health. Staying healthy emotionally and physically also supports your immune system, which is vitally important in cancer treatment.

Talk to your doctor about your sexual concerns. He or she can work with your oncologist to make sure any prescribed treatments are in accordance with your cancer therapy. Bring your partner along as well. It's not unusual for people to worry that cancer might be contagious, or that having sex with someone who is undergoing treatment might negatively affect their partner's health—or even their own. Although these fears are unfounded, it's understandable that you or your partner might be confused or scared, and being able to communicate openly is crucial for both of your sexual enjoyment.

A rarely discussed challenge of long-term disease is that your sexuality often suffers. For many patients, especially after an operation such as a mastectomy, being sexually attractive seems impossible. Your body has changed and you may find that your self-esteem has been damaged significantly. Therapy can help to improve your body image and get back in touch with your sexuality. Some couples might even benefit from sex therapy (see pages 76–77) when making the journey back to a healthy sex life.

Diabetes

Diabetes, an inability to regulate your blood glucose levels, is one of the fastest-growing diseases in the US. Many patients suffer from sexual concerns. In fact, it is estimated that around 75 percent of men and 35 percent of women with diabetes suffer sexual side effects. Not everyone feels comfortable discussing sexual concerns with their doctor, especially if the disease is otherwise well managed.

If your partner has diabetes, he may be suffering from low testosterone (women can also suffer from this). A blood test can help reveal if this is the case. If so, testosterone replacement therapy might be an option (for more on this, see page 247), and there are many other treatments for erectile dysfunction, including medication (e.g. Viagra or Cialis).

Premature ejaculation can also be a side effect of diabetes. If your partner struggles with this, the most important thing is for him to realize that anxiety is one of the key factors. When he gets anxious, the blood vessels in the penis constrict, which compromises the erection. If he loses his erection, focus on sexual play other than intercourse.

Vulvodynia

Vulvodynia, also known as vulvar dysesthesia, is chronic pain in the vulva. This pain can feel like an itching, burning, throbbing, or aching sensation. The pain is generally unexplained and could be due to a number of factors: hypersensitivity to yeast infections; muscle spasms; allergies; hormonal changes; nerve damage; repeated use of antibiotics; or psychological damage due to sexual abuse or trauma.

There are two general categories of vulvodynia. Generalized vulvodynia is not necessarily caused by touch or intercourse. It can occur in different parts of the vulva, and may be constant and frequent or inconsistent and rare. Vulvar vestibulitis involves pain at the entrance to the vagina. The pain begins during intercourse or when touched.

There are many different types of medication used to treat vulvodynia, including nerve blockers, antidepressants, estrogen creams, and localized anesthetics. However, while the absence of pain certainly makes sex better, numbing agents also take away the nerve sensations that make sex so pleasurable. Treatments such as physical therapy and diet modification can help to decrease pain without eliminating sensations.

Embracing your sexuality

With the right modifications and a commitment to open communication, you can embrace your sexuality regardless of disability. The best sexual experience is the one that works for you and takes into account your needs and your desires. Remember that part of the fun of sex is trying new things. Commit to making your sex life the best it can be. See below for ideas on where to start.

First, visit your doctor. Although it might be a little intimidating to broach this topic, the truth is that any good doctor will be aware that sexuality is a crucial part of your health and well-being. If he or she brushes you off or doesn't respond, find a new doctor.

Communicate with your partner. Don't be shy about bringing up any fears or concerns you have about how your condition will impact your sex life. Working through these together can actually make you and your partner grow closer together.

Experiment. If intercourse isn't possible or is uncomfortable, try giving each other a massage, kissing, caressing, or mutual masturbation. Take your time finding out what strokes are erotic for you.

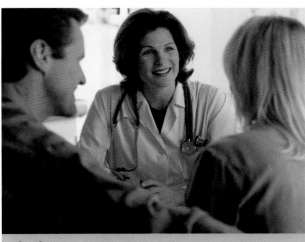

How to...

TALK WITH YOUR DR. ABOUT SEX

Bring your partner along to your doctor's appointment, so that he can ask questions, express any worries, and understand your treatment options.

1 Ask about any issues that accompany your condition, as well as concerns that might arise from having an active sex life. Also ask about safer sex and how to care for your reproductive health.

2 Mention your own unique sexual health needs, and ask about protection that is right for you.

TOP 5

TOP 5 WAYS TO IMPROVE YOUR SEXUAL HEALTH

Committing to improved physical and sexual health will have benefits throughout your life. Your relationship will improve, your intimacy will deepen, and your passion and sexuality will go through the roof. As if that weren't enough, your emotional health—including your self-esteem, your body image, and your overall attitude—will be revamped, too. Read on for the top five ways you can recommit to your sexual health.

1 See your doctor.

If you are having any health concerns, whether it is a recent lack of libido or an ongoing issue such as vaginal dryness or fatigue, then you should speak with your doctor. The medical community is now embracing sexual health as a crucial part of a healthy, happy life, and most doctors are well-versed in common sexual issues and treatments.

2 Talk to your partner.

Open communication is key. You have to be able to talk to your partner about everything from safer sex to reproductive health to mismatched libidos. Sexual health and satisfaction is a direct result of the state of your relationship, so if you are disconnected or dishonest with your partner about your sexual needs, it will affect you inside and outside the bedroom.

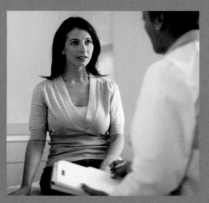

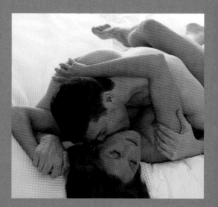

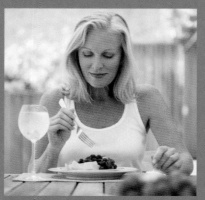

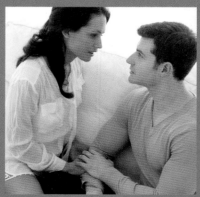

3 Treat your body like a temple.

Make a commitment to respect your body, inside and out. From feeding yourself healthy, nutritious foods to getting active a few times a week, you should make sure that you always make time to care for yourself. Cutting back on caffeine and alcohol, and getting plenty of rest are all part of the TLC that your body needs.

4 Use lubrication and sexual aids.

Don't be afraid to experiment with new things, especially when it comes to making sex more comfortable and enjoyable for you and your partner. Whether it's just to spice things up, or to improve joint and muscle comfort during intimacy, there are a wide variety of sexual aids that can help make your sex life the best it can be.

5 Do your Kegel exercises.

Perform your Kegels regularly to keep your pelvic floor strong and your orgasms intense. To locate the right muscles, squeeze to stop your flow of urine (only do this to find the muscles). Once located, exercise by contracting for five seconds, then releasing for five seconds. You can do this discreet exercise anytime.

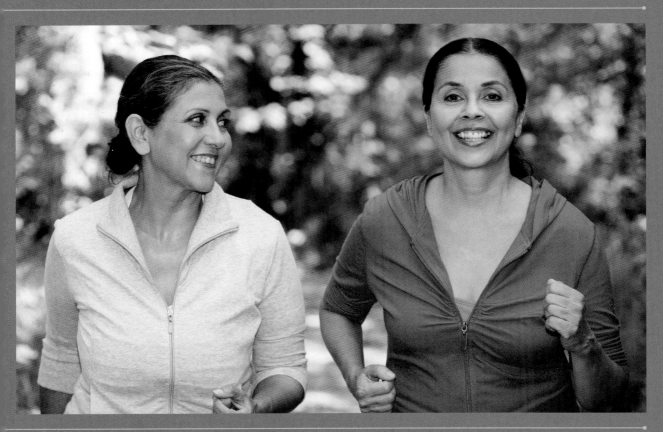

Lovers and caregivers

One of the best parts of being in a relationship is that you know you always have someone you can rely on, through the good and the bad. At times you will be the one who needs nurturing, perhaps when you are ill or going through difficulties with family or at work. At other times, you will be the one in the caregiving role. This trade-off is all part of the give-and-take of a successful, loving relationship.

Dealing with illness

As a woman, you might feel like you slip into the role of caregiver quite easily. Caring for others is an innate female skill. It becomes more difficult, however, when your partner has a long-term illness, because you have to walk the fine line between being his caregiver and being his sexual partner. These roles are difficult to juggle.

If you are the one who is ill, it can be equally difficult to accept care from your partner, especially if you have traditionally been the primary nurturer in the relationship. In fact, it's no wonder that so many couples break up as a result of prolonged illness. It's hard to figure out the new needs and rules of the relationship during this stressful time.

Nurturing your partner

Although illness brings many challenges, there are certain actions you can take to make this period more positive. Throughout, the most important thing is to share your love and keep the peace with your partner in every possible way.

Educate yourself. One of the best ways to learn about your partner's illness is to visit the doctor with him (with his permission, of course). Prepare by making a list of questions to bring with you. You can also take notes about anything relevant, whether it is a recent study or the best time of day for your partner to take his medication. You will be surprised how easily you might forget these details when you are busy acting as caregiver.

Ask for help. Always remember that it's not selfish to ask for help. Taking good care of yourself is the only way you can take good care of others. When you ask someone else to help, be specific and simple in your requests, such as 'Would you mind coming from 4 to 6 PM, so I can go grocery

> **66** It's very important that you own your feelings of sadness or anger and allow them to be expressed. **99**

shopping?" You can also ask for help at times when you are exhausted and simply need to take a nap or get out of the house. Respite care is a good way to find help if you don't have family nearby.

Take advantage of hospice. People often believe that hospice is the last stop before death; however, it can be used long before the patient is dying. If your partner has a terminal illness, a hospice can help with part-time care, sometimes even for a few days at a time. See Resources, page 251, to find out more about hospices, and to find services in your area.

Help your partner to help himself. No one likes to feel incapable or helpless, and this is particularly true for men. It's hard to go from being a strong, capable person to having to ask for help getting out of bed. The effect of sickness on your partner's self-esteem can be devastating. Because of this, it's crucial to try to give him as much independence as possible. Most importantly, don't baby your partner or make him feel like a child. If he says he can do something on his own, let him. You can stand by with a watchful eye in case he needs your help, but try to do so from a distance. No matter how much you might want to help your partner, healing is something he ultimately has to do by himself. By the same token, talk to him and share your thoughts, feelings, and fears just as you always have, rather than trying to hide them. Changing the way you treat him or act around him will only make your partner feel deceived or infantilized.

Appreciate intimacy. Your partner might not be able to have sex, but that doesn't mean you can't be intimate. Stay close by bathing together, cuddling, or even reading erotic stories. It might seem like a time of illness is the wrong time to focus on sexuality, but the truth is that the person is still an adult with sexual thoughts and needs. Embracing these can help reconnect him with his former self.

Allowing grief

One of the most important parts of the caregiving role is to accept and express your feelings of anger, grief, and doubt. You might feel like you shouldn't complain or give in to negative feelings during this time. After all, your partner needs you to be strong. However, the truth is that his illness affects you just as strongly as it affects him. It's very important that you own your feelings and allow them to be expressed, whether you feel fear, grief, depression, anger, doubt, or even loss of faith or denial. People go through a wide range of emotions when someone close to them becomes ill. If you honor those feelings and allow yourself to express them, you will be able to process and work through them, rather than get stuck in your own sadness.

You can speak to a counselor or a faith leader about your feelings, or join a caregivers' network in your own community. Most hospitals have spouse support groups where you can be with others who understand what you are going through. See Resources, page 251, for more information about the stages of grief, and tools that can help.

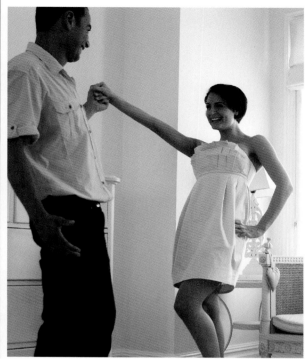
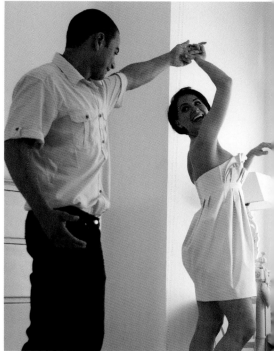

Chapter 5

Being hard to get, not playing hard to get

The master rule that really matters when it comes to finding and keeping the love you want is this: be hard to get. This doesn't mean playing relationship games—it means building a life that is whole, happy, and fulfilling, even when you are single. When you do this, you will be irrisistable to the type of man you want to attract: confident, loving, and looking to build a lasting partnership.

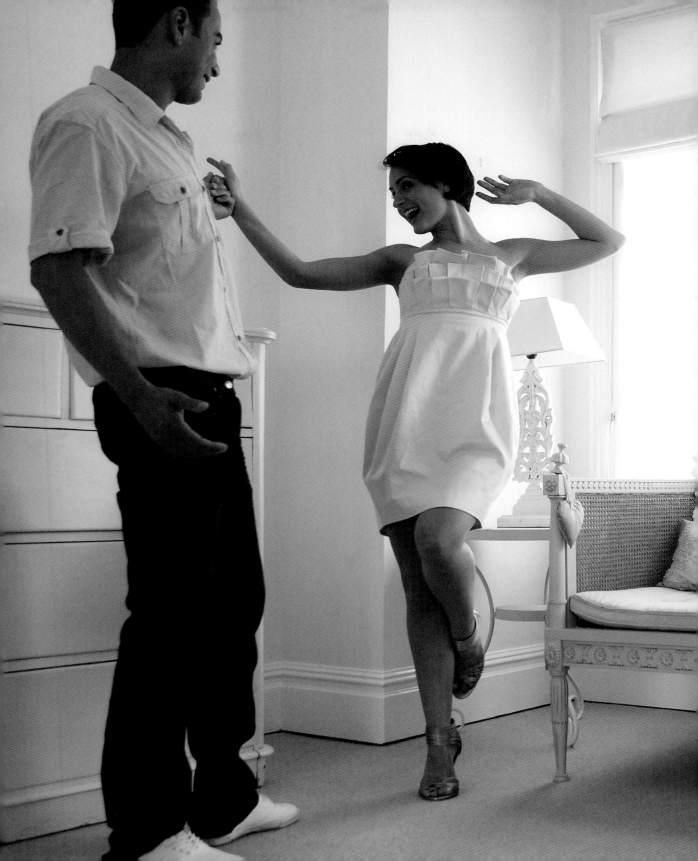

The way you present yourself to the world has a huge impact on the type of people you attract. If you are single, your outlook and attitude are two of the biggest factors in determining what your future relationships will be like. If you are already in a relationship, these same factors will directly influence its success.

Consider these questions, honestly asking yourself how you would respond (not how you think you *should* respond). Then, reflect on what little changes might make you more open and confident.

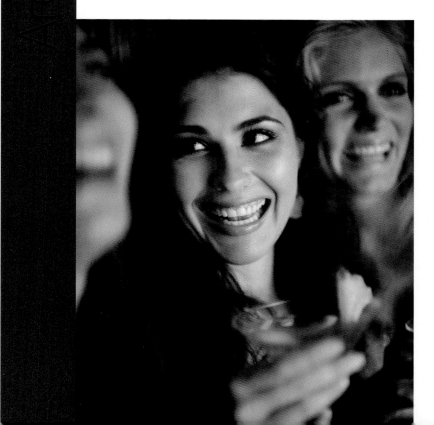

1 YOU AND YOUR FRIENDS ARE HEADED OUT

for a long-anticipated night on the town. At the bar, you see an attractive man checking you out from across the room, so you:

Ⓐ Prowl over to his table and start hitting on him, making sure to get his number before you leave.

Ⓑ Catch his eye, smile briefly, and look away several times until he comes over to you.

Ⓒ Have the waitress send him a drink and your phone number.

2 YOU HAD AN AMAZING DATE ON SATURDAY NIGHT

with a guy you met online. It's now Tuesday. Since the date you have:

Ⓐ Facebooked him, texted him, and sent him several emails covering everything from how much fun you had with him to how work is going.

Ⓑ Not contacted him once.

Ⓒ Sent him a brief text thanking him for a great date.

3 YOU AND YOUR BOYFRIEND HAVE BEEN DATING FOR A FEW MONTHS NOW.

The connection is intense and you guys argue often, usually because he has broken promises or mistreated you. As a result, you:

Ⓐ Whine to your friends that all men are jerks, and obsess over ways you can make him change his behavior.

Ⓑ Go out of your way to make him happy—cooking him dinner, cleaning up after him, loaning him money, etc. Whatever keeps the peace!

C Sit down and have a talk with him about your feelings. If he still mistreats you, you will be out the door.

4 YOU ARE ON VACATION WITH YOUR PARTNER

and are raring to recommit to your sex life. However, your partner evidently didn't get the romance memo, as he seems content to lie in his boxers and watch sports. You:

A Accuse him of being unromantic and thoughtless, and spend the next two hours recounting all the ways he has failed you in the last year and how this has impacted your relationship.

B Behave as if nothing is wrong but silently seethe at him for failing to take initiative once again and for not appreciating you.

C Light some candles, turn on some romantic music, and debut the sexy lingerie you bought for the trip.

5 ON YOUR MORNING COMMUTE, YOU ARE APPROACHED BY A FELLOW TRAIN PASSENGER.

Granted, he is no Brad Pitt, but he seems nice. When he asks for your phone number, you:

A Turn him down. No way are you going to even consider dating someone who is slightly shorter than you when you are wearing heels.

B Give him your phone number and then spend the next few weeks screening your calls and dodging him on the train.

C Agree to meet for coffee. At the very least, you might gain a new friend out of the experience.

6 ON A NIGHT OUT WITH YOUR PARTNER

you notice him casually checking out the bartender. You:

A Ask sarcastically if he'd rather you and she switch places, then continue badgering him playfully but relentlessly when he denies any interest.

B Become very quiet, but deny that anything is wrong when he asks.

C Remember the harmless interest you took in your cute barista earlier that morning and decide the looks mean nothing—but change your conversation to a more flirtatious topic.

7 YOU ARE ACTIVELY LOOKING FOR LOVE.

By active, you mean:

A Initiating contact with every attractive guy you meet.

B Joining an online dating community and hoping your cute profile lures the perfect guy.

C Adding a few new activities to your schedule and asking friends to set you up with any eligible men they know.

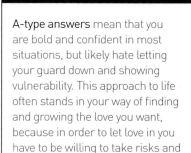

A-type answers mean that you are bold and confident in most situations, but likely hate letting your guard down and showing vulnerability. This approach to life often stands in your way of finding and growing the love you want, because in order to let love in you have to be willing to take risks and open yourself up to others.

B-type answers suggest that you may struggle with insecurity. You might be afraid to own and express your needs, which means that it will be very difficult to be in a relationship where they are met. Instead, you tend to take a passive role in your own life and may let others take advantage of you or avoid taking steps that will secure your own happiness.

C-type answers indicate that you are confident and secure, and that you try to be open-minded. You love yourself and your family and friends, and your positive attitude makes others gravitate toward you. You are in a good place to find and keep a happy, healthy relationship.

66 Your outlook and attitude are two factors that determine what your relationships will be like. **99**

The right way to find love

No doubt you have heard the mantra "Play hard to get." This sisterly advice acknowledges the well-known fact that men like being the pursuer—and further, that men like feeling they are after something special and hard to get. If dating you were an easy feat, it wouldn't boost a man's ego to "win" you in the end.

The science of attraction

It all goes back to the cavemen era. Darwin first introduced the idea, and most scientists and paleontologists agree, that our most basic human drive is to pass our genes on to the next generation. Underneath all the dating games and birth control options and social pressures and romantic negotiation, the imperative to reproduce is inherently present in our DNA.

However, in those cavemen days, it didn't behoove women to mate with numerous men because the risks were too great. A healthy pregnancy was no easy feat back then because pregnancy made a woman increasingly vulnerable and less able to provide food and protection for herself and her offspring, especially during the final months. She needed a good provider, and so she had to be selective. Thus she wanted the strongest and fittest mate, who would not only provide good genes for her offspring, but would also protect and provide for her and the baby in the years to follow.

In contrast, the potential cave-daddies wanted a physically desirable woman to mate with and to support his genes as they were passed on to the next generation. Thus, "desirable" to men basically meant a woman who was what scientists call "reproductively viable"—a very impersonal term meaning that a woman looks healthy enough to become pregnant, survive a pregnancy, and deliver a healthy baby. The cave-daddy was making a big investment in his mate and her offspring. Lots of extra hunting, fighting, and protecting were on the docket during her pregnancy, and really for the first several years of the child's life. He wanted to be sure that the baby was healthy and that it was his. So, if the potential cave-mama seemed like she might be too available, or if she was busy mating with multiple other cavemen, he would move on and look for someone more suited to his needs.

The bottom line? When we strip away social pressures, being hard to get is not a dating game: It's actually in our genes. When you are too easy of a conquest, a prospective partner feels like you're available for any guy, and the relationship won't feel special or secure. He will wonder if you can really be committed and faithful to him.

Avoiding the game

By now, you are probably thinking, "This seems childish. Do I really have to play a game to make a man feel good about himself and want to date me?" Fortunately, the answer is no. The secret is not in playing hard to get, but in being hard to get.

Being hard to get is good for both you and your prospective partner. It isn't about his ego or following the rules of a game. It's about living a full, happy life that satisfies you and enriches you. When you are hard to get, you are confident and secure in who you are, with or without a partner. You have your own life and interests and friends. Of course, you probably still want to meet someone and enjoy love, but you are not going to put your happiness on hold until that happens—and you don't need someone else to "complete" you.

Becoming hard to get

It's easy to spot someone who is hard to get. You know that woman from a mile away, although you might not be sure what it is that is so special about her. On the outside, she appears to be a woman of average looks and sex appeal. However, she carries herself with a style and confidence that has every man in the place checking her out. This confidence has nothing to do with the clothes she is wearing or the stilettos she is sporting. Those are superficial

Defining beauty

In truth, not as much has changed since caveman times as we might think. Men and women today are still attracted by many of the same physical attributes our ancestors gravitated toward, whether consciously or unconsciously. Of course, personality and inner beauty often play equally significant roles in today's dating and mating rituals, but you can't deny that initial physical spark.

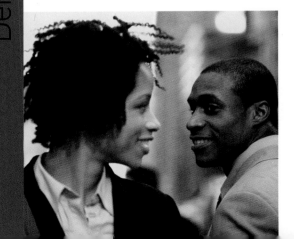

Healthy attraction

Signs of fertility and health are actually the elements we consider beautiful today. These include:
- Symmetrical features
- Smooth, healthy facial skin
- Bright eyes
- Thick hair
- Curvaceous hips

Studies have found that people across the world are attracted to those with facial symmetry, along with a number of the other features listed above. In fact, babies as young as three months old show a preference for people with these traditionally beautiful features, which makes many scientists believe that our preference is actually hard-wired in our brains. This means that attraction is part of the basic human understanding of how the world works.

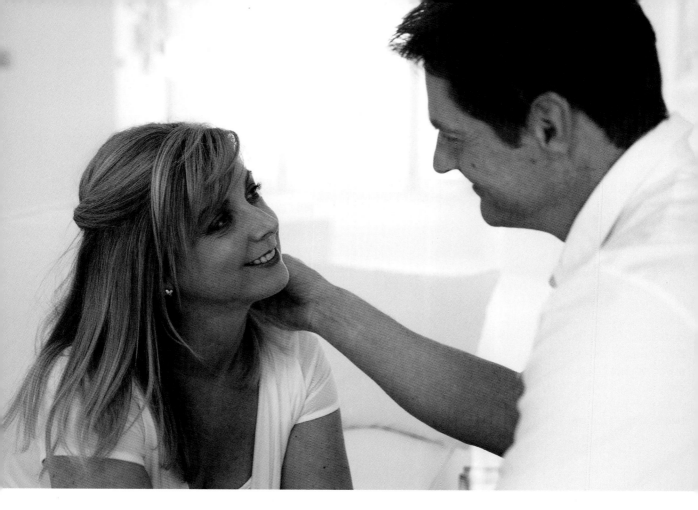

confidence builders. Real confidence comes completely from within, and it can transform an average woman into a potential Hollywood cover girl. Without this confidence, you can land a first date, but you may not get a second. The truth is that you will be unlikely to meet the kind of guys you want to date unless you exude a confidence that draws equally confident people to you.

In fact, being hard to get is equally important once you are in a committed relationship. Married women, listen up! There's nothing sexier than a woman who is confident, independent, and knows her own mind, whether you're on the dating scene or have been married for 20 years. Read on for tips on how to keep this desirable independence at every stage of your relationship life.

Stop pretending, start doing. When you merely play hard to get, you are mimicking a life you want and playing a persona (for more on personas, see pages 226–227). You might pretend to have a busy social schedule or be sexually confident, when really you only have a few friends and have plenty of inhibitions in the bedroom. Instead of continuing to live this charade, try actually funneling that energy into making those changes to your life. For example, if you don't have as many friends as you would like, you could volunteer at a neighborhood soup kitchen or start a book club at your office or plan a block party for your apartment building. There are so many ways that you can meet people and make new friends—but sitting at home pretending to have friends isn't one of them! To follow the second example, if you have inhibitions around sex, think about why that is. Is it because you worry about the way your body looks, or because you had a negative experience with sex in the past? Sharing these feelings with your partner is the only way to true sexual confidence, and you will find that you feel so much better about yourself when you are honest. Being true to who you are is key for all women who actually are hard to get.

Reset your way of thinking. The reason many women struggle with confidence issues is because they are stuck in a negative way of thinking, such as "If I don't meet someone soon, I am going to end up an old maid," or "I bet the reason I haven't met anyone yet is because I am overweight." It is crucial that you find a way to dump whatever negative thoughts you are carrying with you (for more on getting unstuck, see pages 18–19). Until you do, you won't be able to become the woman you want to be. Every woman who is hard to get thinks positively about herself and her attractiveness to others.

Have your own opinions. When he asks where you'd like to go for dinner, the woman playing hard to get will likely say, "Oh, wherever you want" every time. The woman who *is* hard to get is flexible if he has a special restaurant in mind, but she also has a few ideas of her own. A woman who is playing hard to get will spend the whole evening trying to impress her date, whether that means wearing a low-cut, supershort dress or listening enraptured as her date spends two hours bragging about his most recent accomplishments at work. A woman who *is* hard to get will listen to her date attentively, but she will also share interesting and funny stories about her own life, and she will dress seductively, but not in a way that is desperate for attention. Do you see the difference? Women who are hard to get are still alluring, and they still try hard. They simply stay true to themselves in the process.

Show vulnerability. When people play hard to get, they often try to hide their emotions or pretend to have no feelings for the person they are dating. Most women worry that if they show that they like a guy, he'll lose interest. But, as we've established, dating is not a game of winning and losing. When you don't open up to the person you are dating, there is no real spark or passion because you are too busy trying to act light and breezy, instead of real. Although no guy wants to feel like you are desperate or too available, he definitely wants to know you find him attractive and sexy, and that you enjoy his company. Putting your heart out there is a risky business, so if you are acting like you consider your date nothing more than a momentary good time, he will also be afraid to show his feelings, and likely won't take the relationship seriously. Keep your life full with activities and friends that existed before your new love interest came along, but also be honest about how you are feeling.

The truth about...

BECOMING COMPLETE

As much as we all loved the rom-com classic *Jerry Maguire*, the scene when Tom Cruise tells Renée Zellweger, "You complete me" would in real life be a dangerous relationship scenario. It may sound romantic, but in reality it is codependent and unhealthy (for more on codependency, see pages 58–61). Your life partner should contribute to your happiness, but you are the only one who can make yourself complete. Furthermore, there is nothing more attractive to a healthy, confident man than a woman who is complete on her own and is looking for someone to enrich and share her life, rather than looking to meet someone before she really begins living.

The new definition of "sexy"

An undeniably appealing word, "sexy" conjures up different things for different people. In fact, that's part of its charm. Each of us has our own internal script, which dictates what we find sexy and desirable, although confidence, humor, and strength of character are pretty sexy in just about any context.

Abandoning the old definition

There used to be a time when only "bad" girls were sexy. Mothers, wives, and "nice" girls weren't supposed to crave sex or have sexual fantasies. They weren't encouraged to be seductive or confident in their sexual prowess. Only "whores" were wild in bed or liked trying new things in the bedroom. Men even sometimes encouraged these stereotypes by treating their wives like modern-day Madonnas, while having their sexual needs met by girlfriends they kept on the side. After all, men reasoned, the mother of their children deserved to be respected and honored, not to be ravished like a sexual being. Thus, for a long time, these two concepts were mutually exclusive.

This means that there has historically been a lot of damaging language and imagery around the definition of a sexy woman. Many women still struggle with these stereotypes, at least emotionally, no matter how much they know intellectually that "nice" girls can be sexy, too. The idea of putting themselves out there sexually, asking for what they want in the bedroom, and feeling entitled and empowered by their sexuality feels out of their comfort zone, even though a part of them really wants to take control and embrace this special, significant piece of being a woman.

Becoming confident in your sexuality

This is where your confidence can come in. Women don't have to choose between sexual pleasure and motherhood, or between being a 'nice" girl and enjoying sex. Yes, our bodies were built to sustain and nurture life, from pregnancy onward. But our bodies were also built to enjoy sex—in fact, the clitoris has no other physical function beyond giving pleasure. Clearly, we are meant to appreciate sex and embrace our sexual nature, and more and more women are doing this everyday. Many women now realize that their sexual pleasure is just as important as their partner's sexual pleasure, and they aren't in the dark about how to achieve orgasm or how to improve their sex lives.

Working with as many couples and men as I have, it's become quite clear to me that what most engages a man sexually is a partner who is into the sexual act, and is uninhibited and sexually confident. This may seem like a tall order if you are one of the large number of women who grew up learning that sex is wrong or dirty. You may imagine that you'd make a fool of yourself if you tried to talk dirty or prance around in a sexy bustier. But if you try it, you'll realize that it's not as hard as it sounds. Your partner doesn't expect to see a professional stripper in front of him. It's okay not to be perfect. What matters is that you are engaged and having fun (see pages 144–145 for more on letting go of inhibitions).

Dealing with social pressures

Now, what's not sexy? I can sum this up in one word: desperation. Even in today's modern society, plenty of women still feel pressure to find a man and settle down. Our language gives a good indication of why: when older men are single they are "bachelors," but women are still called degrading "spinsters" or "old maids." It's no wonder so many women feel pressured to find Mr. Right.

However, all of this pressure can lead to dangerous desperation. Men are simply not turned on by the scent of desperation (for more on this, see page 51). Additionally, when you operate out of fear, as you do when you are under pressure, you might settle for someone who doesn't meet your needs. In order to get and grow the love you want, you have to be okay with who you are, even when—or especially when—you are alone.

If you are a mother, raising your kids is one of the most important jobs you will ever do. But remember, that is just one piece of you. You are also a sexual being, an erotic woman, and the vixen of your partner's dreams! Don't ditch your sexy side for motherhood— let motherhood enrich you, rather than limit you. Your partner will thank you.

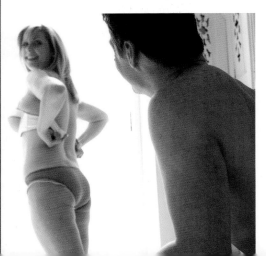

Staying sexy

- **Maintain your interests** Make the transition from mother to lover easier by holding on to your former self. If you make time for friends and hobbies that were part of your life before you had kids, you will be more likely to avoid getting stuck in just one role.
- **Take time for yourself** I've said it before, but I cannot say it enough! Taking time alone to refresh and rejuvenate is crucial to your well-being, and allows you to more easily make the jump to a sexy mindset.
- **Fantasize** It might be difficult at first, but spend some time thinking about what turns you on. The more you think sexy thoughts, the more you will feel like a sexy, desirable woman. That's a promise.
- **Remember, you're a teacher** Your kids need to learn that sex in the right context is good. If you value sex, they will be more likely to value it, too.

Looking for love

You might feel ready to be in a relationship, but if you aren't making that clear to people around you, meeting someone is often much more difficult than it needs to be. Announce to the world that you are looking for love by speaking up and practicing emotionally and physically available behaviors.

Turning your cablight on

Often, the first step to finding love is to turn your cablight on. Coined by Nancy Slotnick in the book *Turn Your Cablight On: Get Your Dream Man in Six Months or Less*, this phrase evokes an important dating truth: When a cab has its light on, people on the street know that it is open for business. If a cabdriver doesn't remember to turn his light on, people forgo flagging the cab down, not realizing that it needs passengers. Take a moment to examine your dating life in light of this philosophy. If you don't have your light on, you aren't going to be approached or asked out, even if that is what you want. Up your dating success rate simply by flipping the switch. You can ensure your cablight is on by following the tips below.

Walk with your head up, make eye contact, and smile. At the grocery store, be friendly with the clerk; at your office, smile at the doorman; at your local coffee shop, chat with the barista. It sounds simple, but these are social cues that everyone around you notices. If Mr. Right is nearby, he will feel much more safe approaching you if he sees you as friendly and open. And even if he isn't in the audience, his friend, sister, or roommate might be. If you make a good impression, you never know where the connection will lead you. Look at every new encounter as an opportunity.

Make confidence matter. You can't be confident if you don't feel good about how you look. Yes, true beauty comes from within, but you won't be your true self, your best self, if you are sitting there feeling glum about the 15 pounds you gained or your bad hair day. Devote time to making yourself feel good by making yourself look good. It's not about being shallow, it's about being confident in your own skin, and that can mean very different

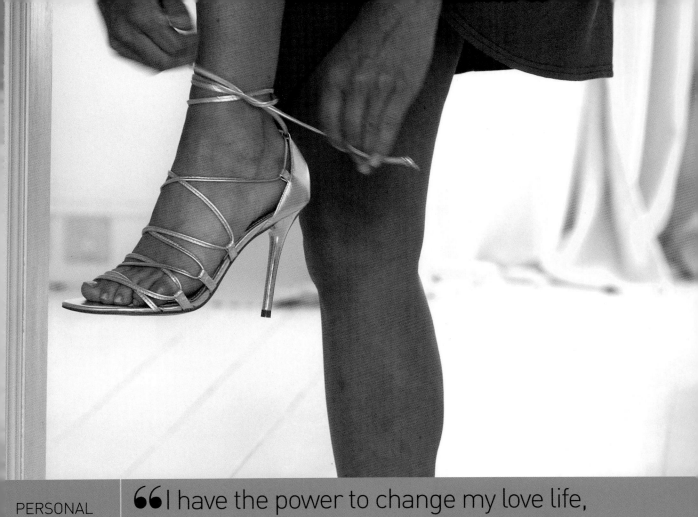

❝I have the power to change my love life, and to attract the right person for me.❞

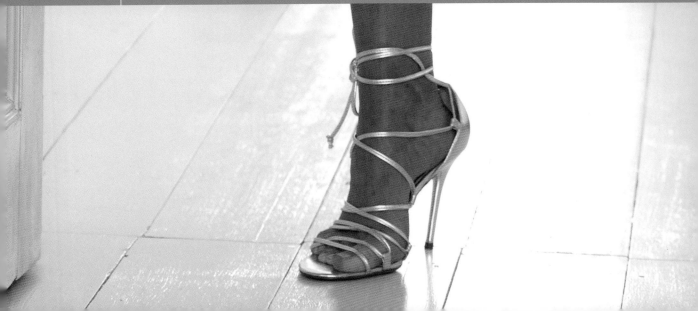

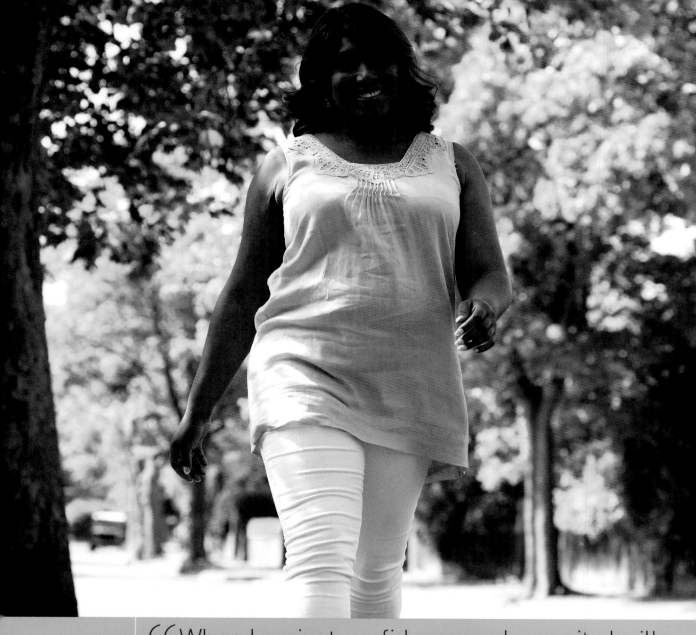

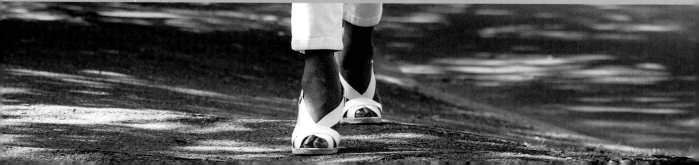

❝When I project confidence and security, I will be noticed and admired by those around me.❞

things to different people. Some women might feel confident with nothing more than a swipe of lipstick and a form-fitting pair of jeans. Others might prefer a touch of glamour, whether that means stilettos, bright highlights, or eye-catching accessories. Whether your style is sporty, classic, modern, or funky, presenting your best face to the world is something you should always make time for—because it makes you feel like you.

Talk to your friends. Sure, your friends and colleagues may know that you are single, but do they know that you are looking? Tell everyone that you are friendly with or comfortable with that you are single and ready to mingle. Ask if they know anyone who might be available, such as a coworker or their boyfriend's friend. You can't just sit on your haunches and wait for love to find you. Plus, meeting someone through a mutual friend is always one of the most comfortable starting points for a successful match. Tell your family as well, and put the word out at your church or temple, or other places where you are involved.

Devote time to your search. You want a fit body? You work out several days a week. You want a successful career? You work overtime to impress your employers. You want to find Mr. Right? You have to put in the same effort that you would toward any other life goal. It seems weird to think of "looking" for love, because people often expect that love will just find them. But if you have gotten tired of waiting for Mr. Right to pop up on your doorstep, it is time to join in on the search. Many experts believe that if you want to find love you have to treat it like a part time job and commit substantial amounts of time—say 15 hours each week—to mingling, dating, and getting out there. Create an online dating profile (for tips on how to do this, see pages 124–125), go to singles' events, and smile and say "hi" to the cute guy on your bus route.

How to...

WALK WITH CONFIDENCE

Think about how you carry yourself, and the energy you are putting out to the world around you. Just like the perfume of desperation (see page 51), people can smell confidence on you, too. Its scent is highly contagious and desirable.

To measure your confidence levels, try an experiment. The next time you are in a crowded area, walk among the crowds in your usual manner. Notice the glances you receive from others, the energy you feel around you, and how your body feels. Then, practice walking with confidence, following the steps below.

1 Pick your head up, lift up your chin, and tighten your transverse abdominal muscles to support and straighten your back (for more information on how to do this, see page 96).

2 Put a little sway in your step, smile (even a subtle Mona Lisa smile works; it doesn't have to be a huge grin), and make eye contact with one or two people that you pass.

3 Notice how different you feel and how differently people react to you. When you check in to the world around you and join it with confidence, you'll find you get a new response. This includes more people checking you out, more smiles back, more confidence in yourself, and more potential dates.

When you set yourself up to look confident, you often start to feel more confident. In fact, this is a useful exercise even if you aren't looking for love. When you carry yourself with confidence, you'll connect more to your inner sensuality, which in turn means you will get a better response from your mate, your co-workers, and just about everyone else in your life.

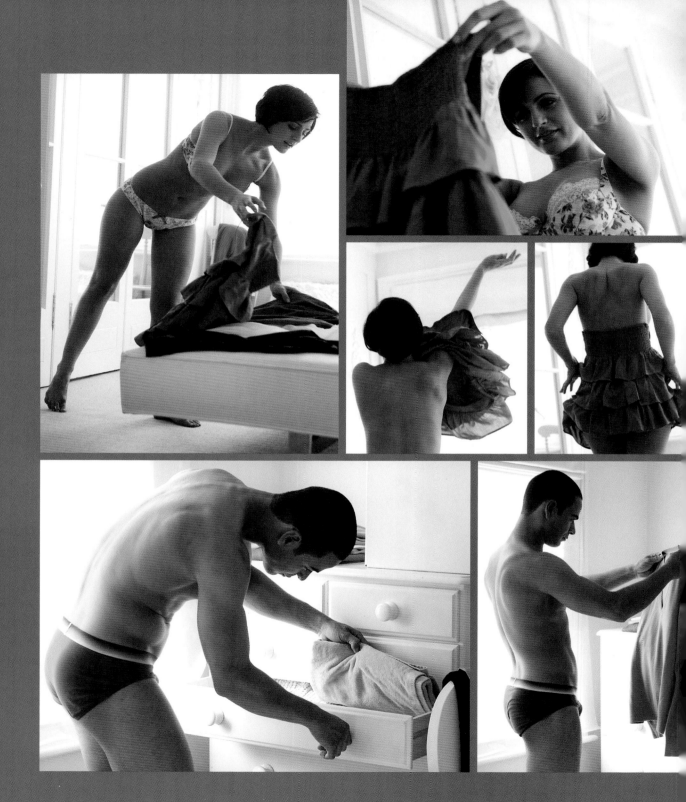

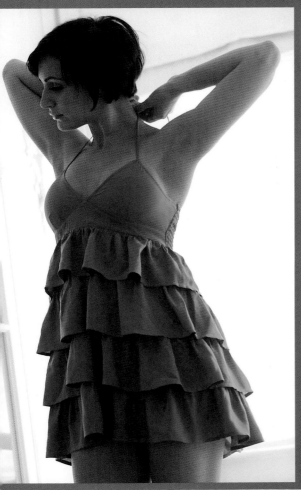

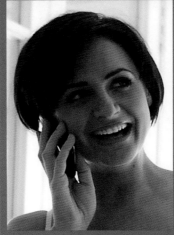

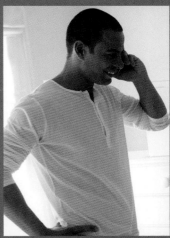

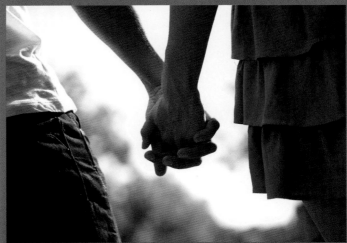

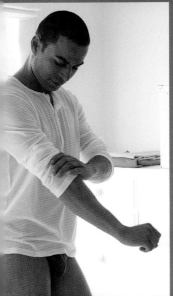

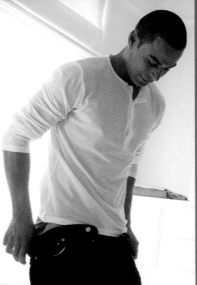

Date Night

Set yourself up for a sensual evening by beginning the flirtation early on. Wearing pretty, playful lingerie will keep you in romance mode from morning to night. Chatting with your date a few hours beforehand will help you stay connected, and will calm any nerves. And choosing a flirty, feminine dress is a foolproof way to start your evening with just the right note of allure.

Internet dating

Online dating can be a great way to meet attractive and interesting singles. Even if you don't meet Mr. Right early on, you will gain more experience in dating and meeting new people, all of which will pay off when do meet "the one." You might have to kiss a few frogs before you meet your prince—but this will only make you that much more appreciative when you finally do meet your match.

Finding the right site for you

If you're struggling to find a dating site, speak with friends or coworkers who have successfully met someone online. Or, search by looking up specific terms, such as "Chicago dating," or "Christian singles." The narrower your search terms, the more likely it is that you will find a site that works for you.

You can also join a handful of sites to see which one matches up with your personality and needs. Most sites have a free trial period, and some are free altogether. Remember that the more sites you join, the more time you will have to devote to maintaining your profiles—but of course, you will also have a higher chance of success.

Standing out from the crowd

The first thing every dating site asks you to do is set up a username or a handle. This is one of the first things people will see when checking out your profile. You want your username to be unique and to reflect something personal about yourself. Think about your name in terms of the image you want to portray and the type of person you want to attract. For example, does HikerGirl, SexyBookLover, or SensualSalsaDancer fit your personality?

Once you've chosen a name and begin to fill out a profile, you will likely be asked questions such as "What is your favorite thing to do?" or "How would you describe yourself?" When confronted with these questions, it is easy to rely on stock answers such as, "I love to shop and go to the beach," but try to be more specific and individual. For example, if you love the beach, you might say: "My perfect day includes a warm beach—and a few unexpected adventures and inside jokes."

The same holds true when you are describing yourself. It is easy to say, "I love to laugh" or "I am smart and I love my family," but descriptions like these aren't very exciting or memorable. Instead, try saying, "I have been told I have an infectious laugh. I have a tough outer shell but I cry like a baby at sappy movies." More detailed anecdotes will set you apart from the crowd and give prospective matches a better idea of what you are all about.

Choosing a picture

Pictures are a must for online dating. If you don't post a picture, daters assume you either aren't who you say you are or that you have something to hide—not the image you want to give off! It's a good idea to post a few different photos. Take one headshot of just your smiling face, then consider adding a full body shot (try to be honest here, no outdated shots from the beach five years ago), and a few pictures of you out having a good time with friends and family. This will show that you are sociable and fun-loving.

Two other things: Try to limit the pictures of you and your pets to avoid giving off a crazy cat-lady vibe, and, if you want a serious relationship, make sure your pictures reflect that. Don't show yourself in anything too revealing, or drinking heavily unless you want to come across as a party girl.

Setting goals

Now that you have your profile set up, don't just sit there! Make it a goal to contact five to ten daters each week. Write a short, flirtatious email to each prospect saying that you saw their profile and wanted to say hello. Mention something specific in their profile that caught your eye, such as their love for the theater or their baseball card collection. Don't make your messages too overtly sexual or over-the-top unless you are just looking for an online hookup. Writing a form email to send to potential dates is a good way to save time, but make sure that each note is a little personal, so that the person knows you aren't just spamming everyone on the site.

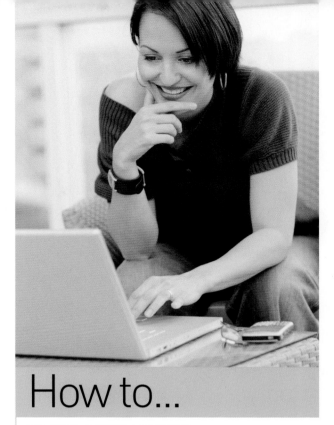

How to...

PUT SAFETY FIRST

So, you have been chatting with HotHandyMan for a few weeks, and decide to meet up. Even if you have spoken with him on the phone and sent each other detailed emails and pictures, that doesn't mean that you shouldn't proceed with extreme caution. Follow these steps to make sure you stay safe.

1 Let your friends know your date's name and when and where you will be meeting. Also, make a plan to send a text message every so often during the date, so that they know you are safe.

2 Meet somewhere public and don't overindulge on the date. A good way to prevent this is to have a coffee date or a lunch date, in which you won't be tempted to linger over wine and go back to his place.

3 If you do want to hook up, take him back to your place instead of going to his, and make sure your friends or family know what's going on.

Overcoming the big dating mistakes

Once you have established that you are looking for love and are actively dating, there are new challenges to face. Getting to know people in a dating environment can be exciting in a way that no other part of your relationship will be—full of promise and spontaneity. To maximize and move forward in this time, however, you must learn to avoid the common dating traps many women fall into.

Seeming desperate

In the dating world, nothing is worse than coming off as too desperate. Maybe your biological clock is in overdrive, or you can't bear to be a bridesmaid in one more wedding without a real date on your arm. But even if you are beautiful, intelligent, and have a great personality, if a guy senses that you are desperate for male attention or commitment, he will sprint in the other direction. Every guy—even those who are seriously looking to commit—is looking for someone who is independent, not needy. This goes back to the male need to feel like he must be special in order to win the prize of your affections.

When you feel desperate, it comes across loud and clear, even if you don't express it verbally. Body language, a sense of urgency, and an overactive desire to please can all be communicated without words. Romance needs space to flourish. If you are forcing a connection you won't have the opportunity to see if there is any potential for longevity.

How do you know if your behavior is coming off as desperate? Brace yourself for useful feedback and ask your friends if your behavior ever seems needy around the opposite sex. Listen to their response, then check out these common "desperate" behaviors to see if you can relate (for additional behavioral clues, read about the perfume of desperation role, page 51).

Dropping everything for him. In the beginning of a relationship, men are hyper-vigilant when it comes to gauging a woman's level of neediness. If a woman suddenly becomes constantly available—he can make plans with her at any time, including 7 PM on a Saturday night, or she's quick to drop her Thursday Girls' Night Out ritual to be with him—he will begin to retreat. Always remember that it is important to maintain your previous interests, whether that is seeing your friends, going to the gym, or giving your all at the office.

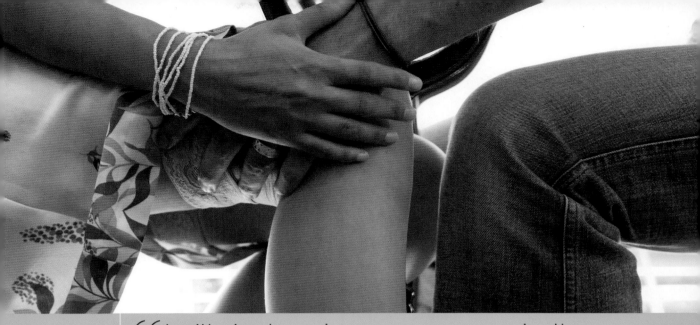

66 I will give love time to grow organically, knowing that I am already complete. 99

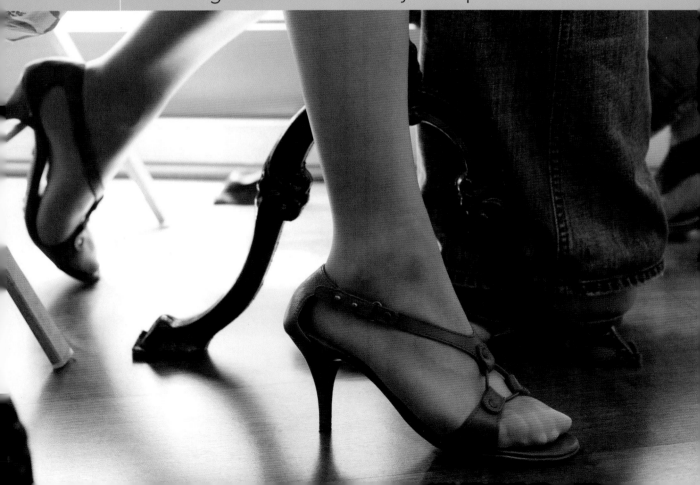

> **66** Sharing emotions is important, but you shouldn't be constantly embroiled in arguments or tiffs. **99**

Overthinking and oversharing. A confident and secure woman can roll with the punches. She doesn't look to a man for validation or completion, so when things go wrong (he is a few minutes late for a date; he hates your favorite movie), she doesn't overthink it or lose her cool. Sharing emotions and communicating honestly are important parts of a relationship, but you shouldn't be constantly embroiled in arguments or tiffs. The beginning of a relationship should be lighthearted and fun, and letting go and enjoying the moment is crucial in showing that you are not desperate for a long-term connection.

Remaining in a rut

Being stuck in a rut comes from being scared—of change, of loss, of regret. If you are stuck in life, you are likely stuck in love. When you live your life in a place of fear, you are in the **Victim** role. This means you see yourself under the control of the situations and people around you. You live in a place of "if only," rather than making proactive changes that will bring you the happiness and satisfaction you seek. This is not a good position for finding love.

If you are single and stuck in a rut, it could be that you find yourself dating the same type of guy over and over again (for more on this, see repetition compulsion, pages 34–37). Or, you might feel like you just aren't making headway into your long-term goal of meeting Mr. Right. The solution might be to make some changes in your life. This could mean completely shaking up your social life, whether it is trying out a handful of new nightlife spots, or joining a singles group at your local parish, or even trying a new grocery store or route home from work.

These simple changes to your lifestyle won't necessarily cause Mr. Right to drop from the sky, but they will give you the opportunity to meet more people, as well as cause you to change your way of thinking. By physically forcing yourself out of a rut, you can create a mental change as well. In addition, you will create a life that is busy and full, which means you will become more and more hard to get.

Being judgmental

Perhaps one of the surest ways to prevent yourself from finding love is by engaging in judgmental behavior. It's okay to hold out for someone who you have chemistry with, but if you make a habit of writing people off at first glance, you will never be able to develop an attraction. Love doesn't always happen at first sight. Sometimes love can begin as a friendship, or even as a business relationship. Being non-judgmental simply means being open to love and accepting of others' flaws and quirks. In fact, finding someone whose flaws you can embrace is what defines love. Loving a perfect man isn't proof of any special connection, but loving an imperfect man is a true testament to your unique bond.

Overcoming the temptation to judge requires a small shift in your way of thinking. For example, instead of deciding, "I want to be with someone rich," think, "I want to be with someone stable and ambitious, who has the same long-term goals as me." Or, instead of thinking, "I want to be with someone who has rock solid abs," think, "I want to be with someone who takes care of himself and is active." Thoughts like these will help you identify the things that are truly important to you, and they will also make you more open-minded, friendly, and attractive toward those around you. (See pages 22–23 for more on rethinking your Mr. Right.)

Struggling with insecurity

Essentially, insecurity is caused by an internal struggle to accept yourself and the world around you. If you aren't emotionally secure and confident in who you are, you are not going to attract people who are good for you. In fact, there is a certain type of guy out there who actually preys upon women who are insecure or weak, as they are easy targets to manipulate. These men may be charming at first, but eventually they might start hitting you up for money or other resources. They may become emotionally or physically abusive, or they may dump you as soon as you have sex with them. The bottom line is that if you are confident and secure, you are going to attract someone who will honor and promote those qualities in your life.

Battling jealousy

In relationships, insecurity often comes across as jealousy—another love killer. We all experience a twinge of the green-eyed monster from time to time, but if you are obsessed with the possibility that your partner is cheating on you, you are going down a path that could result in the ruin of your relationship. Never let feelings of jealousy go unchecked.

Communicating honestly with your partner will help. Try saying, "I know sometimes I go overboard when I accuse you of cheating. It's something I really want to change about myself and it has nothing to do with you." Then, make a genuine effort to change your behavior (for how to change your mindset and your actions, see pages 18–21). Note, however, that this doesn't mean sticking your head in the sand if there is something suspicious going on. Stay aware of what's happening in your partner's life, but also make sure that trust is a part of your relationship. It's foundational.

Dating after divorce

When you date after divorce, your heart isn't the only thing on the line. Between kids, potential step-relations, money issues, and exes, post-divorce dating can be stressful. However, it is an important step to take. When we deny our sexuality and our need for love, we also deny our femininity and our emotional needs, and limit our happiness.

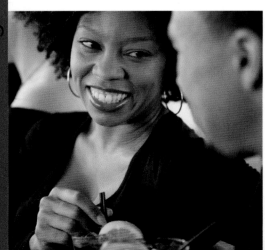

Taking the plunge

● **Know that you will be okay** Reentering the dating world can be scary. You are no doubt afraid of getting hurt again, and maybe you even believe that there isn't someone out there for you. However, the truth is that no matter what happens, you will survive, just like you survived your divorce. Always remember that the chance for reward is worth the risk.

● **Start with Mr. Right Now** Take it slow by accepting date offers from people you only feel "so-so" about. Ease your way back into the swing of dating, and remember: Practice makes perfect!

● **Never discuss your ex** Make this your rule at least until the fourth date. It's okay to briefly mention your divorce, but be careful not to share any negative details. You will come across sounding bitter and desperate—not an attractive early impression.

TOP 10 MOVES TO MAKE ON A FIRST DATE

The best dating advice is just to be yourself, but it can be hard to let your best self come out when dating nerves set in. Here are some tips to help you feel confident and relaxed.

1 Make eye contact.
Eye contact signals that you are confident and interested in your date. Looking around too much will make him think that you are nervous or that you are bored by him. It also prevents you from connecting. Remember that old saying, "the eyes are the windows to the soul"? It's true.

2 Find an excuse to touch him.
Touch him causally when you get the chance. Try putting a hand on his forearm while you laugh at a joke, brushing your arm against him as you walk, putting a hand on his shoulder when you stand up, or touching his back lightly as you walk by.

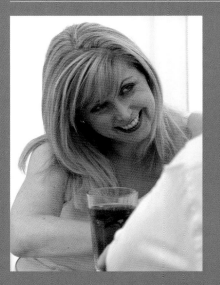 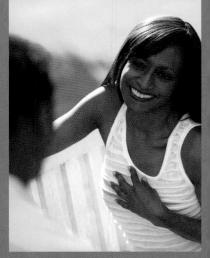

6 Listen.
The attractiveness of listening is highly underrated. Don't let nervousness cause you to ramble off on long-winded stories or share overly personal details. Instead, let him do at least half of the talking, so you can learn about who he is and gauge if there is a connection.

7 Check your body language.
Don't cross your arms or turn your body away from your date, as this can signal that you aren't interested. Instead, turn toward him and mirror his movements. This sends the subliminal message that you are open, receptive, and listening.

It's Not Him, It's You!

How to take charge of your life and create the love and intimacy you deserve

Laura Berman PhD

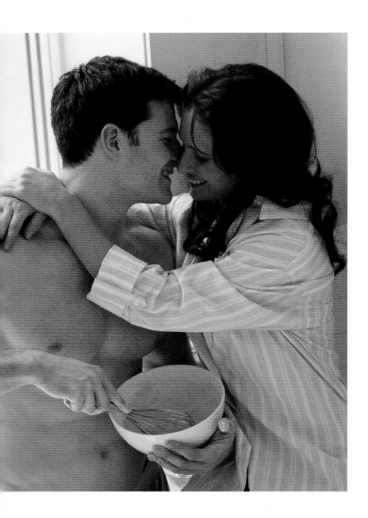

Contents

Dedication

This book is dedicated to my mother, Linda Berman, who recently left this world but will never leave my heart. I didn't think I could survive without you, and it's only due to the perspective and strength you taught me along the way that I've been able to do so. You modeled for me what it is to be an empowered woman, a generous wife, and a dedicated mother. You'll always be my inspiration and I'll always be trying to do it all as well and be as joyful as you along the way. I know you are somewhere smiling and cheering me on.

Getting the love you want

We all want the perfect relationship. Since childhood, we have learned about soul mates, destiny, and happily ever after, and we want those early fairy-tale dreams to become a reality in our adult lives. Unfortunately, we assume this idealized relationship will come to us simply and easily, just as it does in our favorite childhood tales or in the movies we watch over and over again.

Then, when Mr. Right doesn't fall into our laps, or our relationships don't pan out in this idyllic manner, we become disillusioned and angry. We look for someone or something to blame, whether it is our partners, our jobs, or the entire male species. Unfortunately, placing the blame on others does nothing to improve our relationships. Instead, it acts as a toxic force that prevents us from taking control of our lives and finding the love, sex, and intimacy we so want.

The first step in doing this is to put away blame and step into your own power. Only then are you able to change your life in the ways you long to do. In contrast, when you point the finger of blame at yourself, your environment, your situation, or your significant other, you are stuck. You can't make the changes you want, and you can't attract positive people into your life. When you are stuck in a negative and unproductive mindset, all of that pessimism follows you like a dark cloud, poisoning your relationships and preventing you from getting and growing the love you want. My goal in this book is to give you the tools to stop the negative cycle that we all get stuck in from time to time, and help you take control of your love life.

In the following pages, you will learn how to let go of blame and initiate necessary change, how to embrace your own power without always having to be in control, and how to create all the love and intimacy and joy and sex you long for—all by yourself. If you follow my advice, I can promise you will feel safer and clearer and more powerful than you imagined. You will have more romance, more spontaneity, and more passion, along with improved communication and self-esteem.

Each chapter will teach you different tools to help you get and grow the love you want. First, you'll learn how to identify the toxic blame games that trap you, and how these can prevent you from picking the right mate or maintaining a healthy relationship. Then, you will discover how your past might be playing a role in your present love life, and how to break unhealthy dating and relationship patterns that you might not even know you have. From there, you will learn to start creating the emotional and physical changes you want, whether you're hoping to build a stronger connection with your partner, manage maternal guilt, or simply make your daily life more sensual and fulfilling. You will discover how to be fully present in life and in relationships in a way that empowers both you and your partner. And, you will learn how to inspire your partner to be more attuned and connected to you, and to give you the love and intimacy you deserve.

In this book, you will also learn how to take the reins of your own sexual pleasure and create the romance and passion you crave. From intimate new positions to erotica and sex toys that spice up your bedroom routine, the techniques you'll learn are guaranteed to make your time in the bedroom a lot more exciting. Most importantly, you will learn that you don't have to sit around and wait for a great sex life to sprout up overnight. You can plant these seeds yourself.

Every happy couple has one thing in common—they know that they have to work to keep their bond strong and their passion sizzling. The more you work at your relationship and spend time creating the love you want, the more naturally it will happen. The most important step is getting over the idea that great relationships are effortless, or that the perfect man will simply drop into your lap. The second most important step is realizing that your partner can't be responsible for making your relationship change, nor can he read your mind and simply give you what you want. Only you can do that. Keep reading to learn how to create and maintain the love you want. All you have to do is open your mind and come along for the ride!

XO

Laura Berman

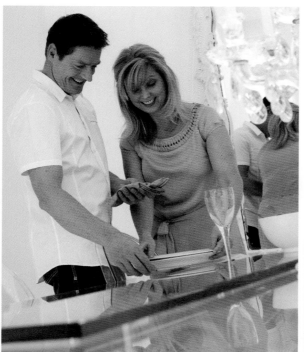
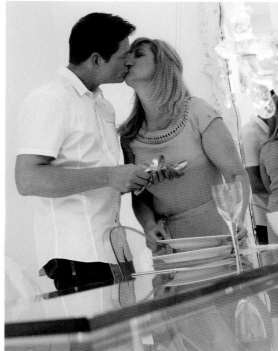

Chapter 1

The blame game

We all seek to blame everyday—fixating on the actions of others, as well as on any number of factors outside of our control. This type of thinking prevents us from feeling content and at peace in every part of life, but particularly in our relationships. It is only when we choose to stop blaming and to take responsibility for our own happiness in life and love that we are able to build the passionate, intimate, fulfilling partnerships we all desire.

3 Compliment him.

Not in an overly exuberant way, but try complimenting his tie, his conversation, his wit, even his attractiveness. Just like us, every man likes to feel attractive and admired. When you do this, you will be expressing your interest in an appropriate and un-needy way.

4 Touch or play with your hair.

Try subtly touching your hair during your conversation. This gives off a sensual cue, and—consciously or unconsciously—will make him think of touching your hair himself. You can also touch your collarbone as you talk, or lightly massage your neck.

5 Remember to smile.

Projecting a positive and happy disposition is key, so don't forget to smile often throughout the night, even if you are nervous. This will also make it clear that you are enjoying yourself. Also, don't forget to laugh when appropriate. Men love a woman who appreciates their sense of humor.

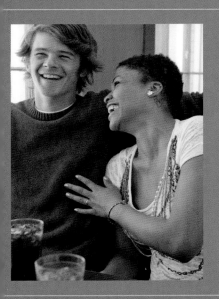
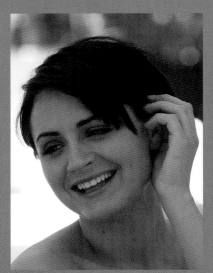
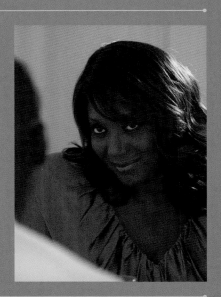

8 Avoid talking about past relationships.

On the first few dates, it is best to avoid any horror stories about past failed relationships. No one is attracted to bitterness. Showing your anger about past loves will only make your date wonder how you will talk about him when the night is over.

9 Be sensual.

Want a foolproof way to guarantee a second date? Order a martini and then take your time nibbling your olive off the skewer, or slowly and seductively eat the cherry off your dessert. Let him see that you aren't afraid to be sexy, even in the middle of dinner.

10 Play up your assets.

Don't show off everything, but choose one asset to draw his attention to, such as your great legs or your toned arms. By showing off just the right amount of skin, you will get his attention and create the right level of seduction without seeming desperate.

Dating and sex

The issue of intimacy timing in a new relationship is a common concern to those in the dating world. Women wonder: "How soon is too soon? I want to be perceived as hard to get, but I don't want him to think I'm a prude!" You can minimize concerns like these by keeping communication channels open, and by being honest with both yourself and your partner about your needs and the level of trust in the relationship.

The right time

Although plenty of people—women and men alike—try to weigh in on the "right" time for two people to begin having sex, the truth is that only you and your date will know the answer to that question. Certainly, having sex on a first date can be a death knell if your partner decides that a one-night stand is all he is after. On the other hand, many happy couples broke that rule of no sex on the first date and have been together for years. The truth is there is no easy answer, and what works for one couple might not work for another. You must take both of your desires and beliefs about sex into account when setting your sexual timeline.

Learning about these sexual beliefs and desires is an important part of the dating process, but perhaps one you don't want to delve into until you know each other better—one reason why first-date sex can be too early. Ultimately, you should only have sex when you feel comfortable with the idea, and when you and your date have discussed past sexual histories—at least as far as STD testing goes—along with safer sex options, including methods of birth control and condom use. For more resources on STDs and birth control, see page 251.

Examining what you want

Some women become so nervous about the first night with a new partner that they overindulge in alcohol and rush into sex. If a one-night stand is what you want and you are practicing safer sex, feel free to explore. However, if you are trying to get and grow good love, it isn't likely that random sex is truly what you desire. If you are looking for real love, you have to make sure that you are taking your most important needs into account, not just your immediate sexual needs. (Remember, now that you have read about self-stimulation on page 106, you can take care of your sexual needs after the date!)

Very few women can have sex without becoming at least a little bit attached. This is because, when we reach orgasm, our brains become washed in oxytocin, the "attachment" chemical, creating a sense of bonding and intimacy. This is true even if we don't really like or know the person we're with. Because of this, I recommend that you don't have sex with someone you don't want to fall in love with, as this can lead to frustration and heartbreak.

Instead of focusing on what you imagine his expectations are, listen to your heart and have sex when you are ready, whether it is on the third date, the fifth date, or the twentieth date. Personally, I am a big fan of waiting to have sex until you are both ready to be in a monogamous relationship, both for protection of your heart and for protection from STDs. You are the steward of your body and your sexuality, and you have the responsibility to treat it well. If you don't, no one else will!

Hesitations about first-time sex

As excited as you are to take this leap of intimacy, most of us have some hesitations with a new partner. What if he isn't attracted to you? What if he does something you don't like? What if it's awkward, or there is no spark? Thankfully, if you wait enough time before becoming intimate, questions like these will probably already have been answered. This is just one of the many benefits of postponing sex until you know your date better.

Yet no matter how comfortable you feel, the first time is always a bit intimidating. That's okay. Admit to your partner that you feel nervous and that you want to take things slowly. If something happens that you don't feel comfortable with or don't like, speak up. And remember, don't put too much emphasis on the first time. Give yourself time to get to know each other's bodies—and have fun!

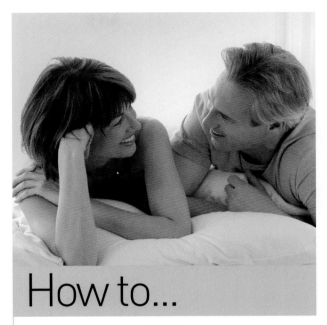

How to...

TALK ABOUT STDS

Discussing STDs with your partner can be a little embarrassing, but it's vital that you do this, for your sake and his. On your third date or so, before you have sex, but when you know you are attracted to him and things are going well, it's time to bring it up.

1 You can be a bit humorous about it. Consider saying something like, "You know, I only discuss my sexual history with people that I am interested in. Since this is getting pretty interesting, I think we should talk about getting tested for STDs."

2 Next, tell him when you last got tested (for more on where to get tested for STDS, see page 251).

3 You can even suggest that the two of you get tested together. Remember: If you are mature enough to have sex, you are mature enough to take this step.

Being hard to get in a relationship

If you're already in a relationship, you might have read this chapter and breathed a sigh of relief that your days of struggling to put forth just the right degree of availability are in the past. However, the truth is that it is just as important for those in a long-term relationship to practice being hard to get. This behavior is one of the best ways to keep the attraction and momentum alive in your relationship.

Monitoring information sharing

Many women go home at the end of the day and spend the next two hours filling their partner in on everything that happened at the office or at the kids' school or on the phone with their mother. Every single detail of your day gets hashed and rehashed, just as it would if you were talking to a close girlfriend.

This type of communicating reflects a basic and often misunderstood difference between men and women. Men typically like to hear the main point first, with just a few details filling in the blanks afterward. Women generally enjoy starting with the details, and eventually getting around to the main point. The problem is that you often lose your partner along the way if there are too many details. It's certainly okay to fill him in on the main events of your day, but it's often smart to save the minute details for your girlfriends. Remember that the man in your life simply may not want to know about your coworker's funny imitation of your boss, or whether you had a chance to buy new tights at the store.

It is also a good idea to be careful not to give too much information about less than attractive incidents. Think back to your early days of dating—you would never have dreamed of telling him that you had a stomachache and gas after lunch. Trim the "fat" off your conversation by only giving him the juiciest and most interesting tidbits of your day. Then, sit back and let him do some of the talking (for more on speaking a man's language, see pages 180-181).

Encouraging his pursuit

I often urge women to take charge of their own sexual pleasure and make the changes they crave in their relationship. For example, if you want more sex, initiate it. If you want more spice, be bold and try something new. However, there are also times when you need to let your partner pursue you. The idea is that you wave him in, but let him do the landing.

You know your partner best, so it won't be very hard for you to get his engines going. Maybe you give him a pat on the behind and tell him he's looking sexy. Maybe you change clothing in front of him, showing off some sexy new lingerie, then casually ask if he'd like to open the bottle of wine that's chilling in the fridge. When you are relaxed and sexy, but aren't openly initiating sex, it will drive him crazy, just like in the first days of dating when he wanted to make a move, but wasn't sure if he should.

> **66 You know your partner best, so it won't be very hard for you to get his engines going. 99**

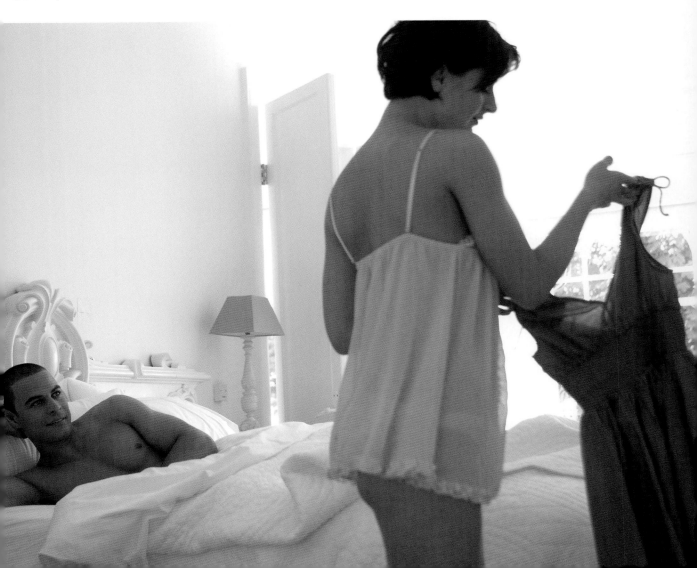

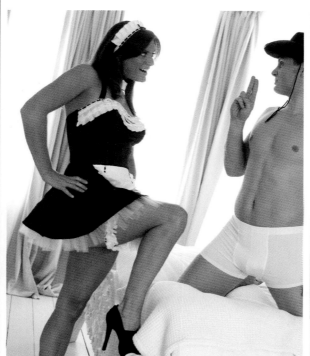
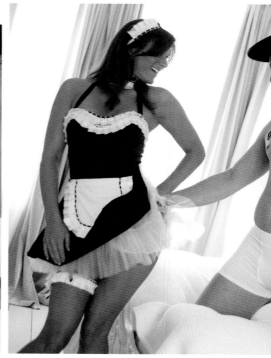

Chapter 6

Unleashing your inner vixen

Every woman has a vibrant vixen inside that is just waiting to jump start her love life. To release this sultry power, all you have to do is rethink the way you value sex. In fact, you can turn a good relationship into a great relationship—or a bad relationship into a good one—simply by committing to work at your sex life, renewing intimacy, passion, and romance along the way.

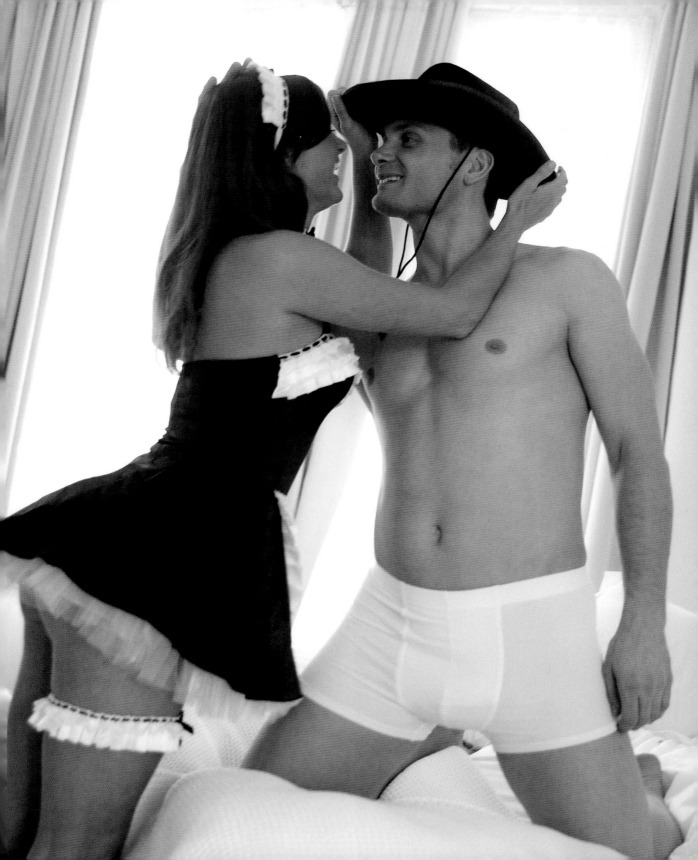

A vixen is a woman who is confident, happy, and inherently sexy. She knows what she wants and what her partner wants—and how to get it. As a result, her relationship stays passionate and exciting, and also secure.

Honestly answer the following questions to help identify where your own inner vixen rules, and where you might need to add a little more oomph to your outlook. Then read on to learn how to create a love and sex life that is romantic, passionate, and full of true vixen appeal.

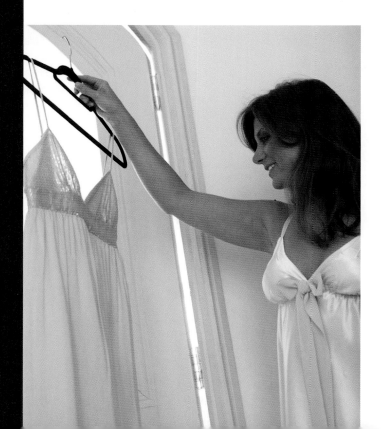

1 IT'S SATURDAY NIGHT. YOUR PARTNER WANTS TO KNOW what you want to do for your weekly date night. You tell him:

Ⓐ "Oh, whatever you want. I guess dinner and a movie is fine. Should we try our usual Italian place?"
Ⓑ "Let's try that new Middle Eastern restaurant downtown. I hear they have great food, live music, and dancing!"
Ⓒ "I'm not sure," then shrug your shoulders and wonder why you always have to plan everything.

2 YOU HAVE A BLACK-TIE WORK FUNCTION on Friday night. After some debate, you decide to wear:

Ⓐ Your usual black shift dress with pumps instead of flats. That should be appropriate, but still comfortable.
Ⓑ A form-fitting dress and a sexy new bra that adds a cup size. (Just having it on under the dress makes you feel sexier!) It's been awhile since you've had a chance to put this much effort into the way you look.
Ⓒ The dress you wore to your sister's wedding two years ago. You hate it, but it's better than spending money on a dress for a work event where you don't really have anyone to impress.

3 YOUR PARTNER JUST GOT A BIG PROMOTION AT WORK. To celebrate, you:

Ⓐ Take him and the kids out for steak and seafood downtown.
Ⓑ Send the kids to your sister's house and spend two hours cooking dinner and turning the bedroom into a sexy

retreat. You know he will be blown away by the effort—even if the chicken is a little rubbery!

C Give him a peck on the cheek and tell him congratulations, then go back to folding the laundry. The house is a wreck and you have a million things to do before you even think about celebrating together.

4 YOU AND YOUR PARTNER ARE GETTING INTIMATE
when he suddenly loses his erection. How do you respond?

A Assume it's your fault and ask him self-consciously what you did wrong.

B Help him become aroused again by doing that thing with your tongue that he loves so much.

C Take it as a sign that tonight just isn't the night, and then immediately roll over and go to sleep.

5 YOU HAVEN'T HAD AN ORGASM DURING
intercourse in a long time, so you:

A Fake it! You would never want your partner to feel badly.

B Tell your partner you want to try a new position that gives you more stimulation, and then hop on top and show him what you're thinking.

C Tell your partner that you just aren't in the mood. If you don't get to orgasm, why should he?

6 YOU GET INTO A SMALL ARGUMENT WITH YOUR PARTNER ON THE FIRST DAY
of your annual anniversary vacation. How do you respond to this setback?

A You feel a little hurt, but honestly expected this to happen at some point during your trip. You and your partner have both been tired and busy lately. You'll patch things up later.

B You decide you both need some space, so go take a walk on the beach for an hour. When you get back, you change into a sexy sundress and order up some cocktails to help you both get back into vacation mode.

C You try to forget what happened, but can't seem to put the argument behind you. It might have been over a small issue, but surely it signals something larger. Things like this never seem to happen to your friends—or on television!

7 AFTER 10 YEARS, YOUR SEX LIFE IS GETTING A BIT STALE.
You decide to:

A Focus on all the other positive things about your relationship. No one can expect to maintain passion forever.

B Start wearing lingerie on a more regular basis, and buy a couple of sex toys as a surprise for your partner.

C Remind yourself that your figure has changed, so your sex life can't be expected to stay the same.

A-type answers mean that you have hesitation or anxiety about unleashing your inner vixen. Although you love your partner and treat him well, you have not fully shown him your powerful, sexual side. This may be because you have a hard time believing that sex is truly an important and meaningful part of a happy long-term relationship. Until you reconnect with your inner vixen you will likely struggle to increase the passion in your relationship.

B-type answers indicate that you are well acquainted with your inner vixen and are comfortable with your own sexuality. Good for you!

C-type answers suggest that you have become disillusioned and doubtful of your own sex appeal. You likely don't believe that you have an inner vixen, and you don't want to run the risk of looking foolish for trying to tap into your sexy side. Your low expectations for life and love often cause you to feel unhappy. In this cold climate, your inner vixen cannot thrive or be powerfully present in your relationship.

66 A vixen knows what she wants and what her partner wants—and how to get it. **99**

Taking the reins of your sex life

Stepping up to take control of your sex life can sound daunting, but it is truly key to your happiness and fulfillment in a relationship. Being in charge doesn't mean initating sex every single time or becoming a domineering, porn-star style lover. It simply means understanding what brings you pleasure, becoming comfortable with a little seduction, and sharing the responsibility for your sex life with your partner.

The female vixen

What is a vixen? If you look at the early definition of the word, it meant two things: a) a female fox, or b) a "quarrelsome" or "malicious" woman. My modern definition of "vixen" is sort of a combination of both of these meanings. Most people picture a vixen as a traditionally sexy woman, complete with red lipstick, sky-high stilettos, and big, bombshell hair. However, for me, a vixen is more than this. She is a woman who is a little naughty. She is bold, connected to her sensual side, and not afraid to seduce her partner. She is not quarrelsome or malicious, but she is also not a shrinking violet. This is not a woman that you would describe as "cute." She's much sexier than that.

For many women, the idea of being anything other than "cute" can be daunting. Most of us were raised to be nice girls, girls who say please and thank you, and never raise their voice or ask to be first. Not only does this prevent us from getting what we desire in life, it also prevents us from getting what we desire in the bedroom. When we don't acknowledge our inner vixens, our needs will not be met, and neither will the needs of our partners. Believe it or not, men don't really want "cute" in the bedroom. It's okay if you still cry at sappy movies and like stuffed animals, but that's not what men want when it's time for intimacy. Although men sometimes like to take control, they may also like to be intimate with a woman who is a little greedy, a tad voracious, and completely comfortable with her sexual desires.

The vixen transformation

Even if you realize that it's good to be a vixen in the bedroom, you might still think it's not for you. You might reason that you aren't a sexy pinup, you haven't painted your nails ruby red since junior high, you don't own a stitch of see-through lingerie, and you feel completely intimidated by the idea of taking charge in the bedroom. You might think that you're not desirable enough, or that you are not deserving of sexual pleasure until you lose 5, 10, 15 pounds. You might abstain from wearing lingerie or sexy clothes because that's just "not you." You might imagine your partner would laugh at you or think it ridiculous if you tried to seduce him. All too often, women think all of these things.

But guess what: These thoughts are not true! While not every woman enjoys fake eyelashes or stilettos, every woman has a sexual, adventurous side. The problem is that it often gets buried under to-do lists, family responsibilities, work commitments, and insecurities. In order to unleash your inner vixen, you have to find a way to release yourself from tedious worrying and get into a sexy, happy frame of mind. Here's how.

> **❝** A vixen is bold, connected to her sensual side, and not afraid to seduce her partner. **❞**

Put your own oxygen mask on first. As anyone who has ever been on an airplane knows, you have to put your own oxygen mask on before you can effectively help others. In other words, if you aren't in a healthy and secure place, you can't be of use to the people in your life who need you. This is why taking time to take care of yourself is so important.

What is a vixen?

Every woman has her own internal definition of what "vixen" means. Men do, too, for that matter. Yet while the specifics of "vixen" can change from person to person, the following truths are part of the heart, mind, and soul of every vixen. Use them to help your own passionate, vixen-like power grow and flourish.

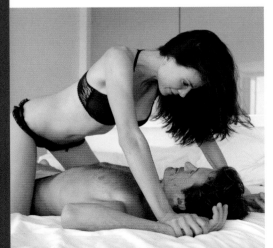

A vixen:

- **has a powerful sexuality** and integrity.
- **is a seductress** in the bedroom and beyond.
- **stays in touch** with her deepest desires.
- **is comfortable in her own skin** and adores and cares for her own body.
- **is unashamed** of her sexual needs and speaks up about them.
- **does not allow society's taboos** or stereotypes to dictate her sexual desires.
- **faces her own demons** and overcomes her own negative feelings about sex.
- **is creative in the bedroom** and shares an active fantasy life with her partner.
- **does not wait for her partner** to initiate sex.
- **has a fulfilling, passionate love life** that is recharged through sexual intimacy.

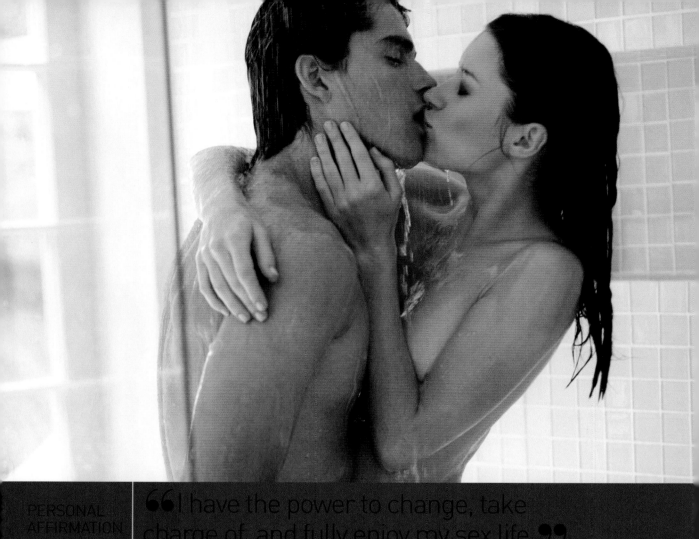

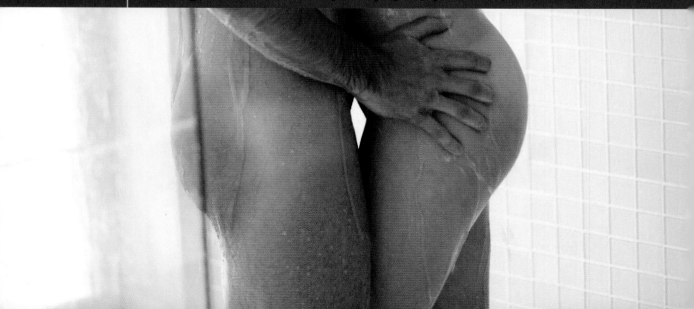

"I have the power to change, take charge of, and fully enjoy my sex life."

It's not selfish to want to devote time to your relationship or your sex life. It's not selfish to want to enjoy how you look and feel good about yourself. Taking 30 minutes to meditate or an hour to go to the gym does not a bad person make!

This is an especially important lesson for mothers. Taking time for yourself means that you are teaching your children valuable lessons about how to present themselves to the world. A woman in touch with her inner vixen takes time for herself because she realizes we all need time for ourselves. Without it, we are too energy-deficient to enjoy our lover and our sexuality, and we miss out on the joy of discovering all the possibilities of who we are sexually and otherwise.

Keep up appearances. Love is certainly more than skin deep, but part of the reason your partner married you was because he was attracted to you. Attraction and desire are an undeniable part of any romantic relationship. No one expects you to look like you did 20 years ago on your wedding day, but you can still make an effort to look and feel your best. That means that even though you'd rather hang around the house in a holey t-shirt, sweats, and your favorite socks, it sometimes serves to try wearing something comfortable, but at least suitable for going to the grocery store.

Make your appearance a priority in a new way—your partner will notice. This might be as simple as throwing out your granny panties and wearing some bright, form-fitting boy shorts. Or, maybe you need to update your hairstyle or purchase new makeup. When you put an effort into your appearance, not only does your partner find you more attractive, it's also a clear sign to him that you care about yourself, your relationship, and his attraction to you—all things that are crucial to his sense of desire and connection with you.

Learn to create your own sexual pleasure. You can't rely on your partner to hold the key to your sexual satisfaction. A vixen is able to enjoy and explore her own sexual desires, whether she is single or in a relationship. The more you become attuned to your own sexual pleasure, the more you will enjoy sexual activity with a partner, and the more comfortable you will feel.

Often, when women have sex, they wonder "Do my thighs look huge?" or "Does it smell weird down there?" or "Am I making strange noises?" All of these thoughts can prevent you from being able to reach orgasm and fully enjoy sex with your partner. Self-stimulation can help you become comfortable with your body and sexual response—and the more you "practice" enjoying pleasure, the easier it will be to reach orgasm with your partner. (For more on how to self-stimulate, see pages 106–107.)

Make time for your partner. Connecting with your partner beyond the bedroom makes it a lot easier to get into the vixen mindset. Choose a ritual that is meaningful for you, whether that means enjoying a glass of wine before dinner or taking a shower together before work or simply cuddling for a few moments. Taking 30 minutes a day to enjoy each other's company in an adult way can do more for your libido than all the lingerie in the world.

> 66 The more you become attuned to your own sexual pleasure, the more you will enjoy sex. 99

Thinking like a vixen

Thinking like a vixen is the first step in learning to act like one. In fact, you can't do one without the other. Of course, sometimes it's easier to focus on mundane everyday tasks than on passion and romance—but the good news is that with practice and purpose you can train yourself to do both.

Changing your thought process

It's not unusual for women to struggle going from "mommy" to "naughty." In fact, some women have a hard time going from "employee" to "naughty," or even "wife" to "naughty." We get caught up in our daily responsibilities, whether that's changing diapers, cooking dinner, leading board meetings, or caring for elderly parents. And it's very hard to feel sexy when you are stressed out, you haven't shaved in a couple of days, and the kids are making a mess somewhere just down the hall.

The key is to get out of your head. It sounds simple, but it requires a bit of practice. Unhooking from the daily whirlwind and enjoying your partner isn't always easy, but the more you do it, the better you will get at it. Before you know it, you will be able to think vixen-like thoughts just as easily as you can think like an employee, wife, mother, and friend. Here's how to start:

Learn to quiet your mind. Take a few minutes to sit quietly, breathe deeply, and come back to yourself. If you feel silly sitting cross-legged and chanting "om," then try a few relaxing yoga positions, or listen to some soothing music with your eyes closed. Find out what works for you, whether that is writing in a journal or retreating to your backyard to sit in a swing and commune with nature. By grounding yourself and coming back to your essence, you can shut out the rest of the world, and have an easier time tapping into your sexuality.

Accept that life isn't perfect—and neither are you. So the house is a little messy and you are badly in need of a pedicure. You can't wait until your body, your house, or your relationship is "perfect" to enjoy your sexuality (for more on "living in the now," see page 81). If it helps, simply fantasize those flaws away, or try envisioning yourself as a bold, sexual goddess who isn't held down by such earthly concerns. This will help you learn to enjoy sex, regardless of whether you are at your ideal weight or have a home that could be featured in a magazine. Embracing your flaws and your partner's flaws is what real relationships are all about.

Thinking sensually

The more in touch you are with your senses and your sensuality, the more tuned in to your inner vixen you become. Make it a point to focus on all of your senses every day. This may mean walking slowly down a sidewalk and taking time to notice the soft breeze and the feel of sun on your skin. Or, it may mean eating more slowly and sensually (for more on this, see page 91). These are easy ways to stay conscious and connected to your senses—and the more in touch you are with your senses outside the bedroom, the more in touch you become inside the bedroom. If you are still having trouble feeling or acting sensual, try the tips below.

Notice your partner. Be purposeful about enjoying your partner's presence the way you did when you were first dating. There are lots of little ways to do this. Try nuzzling his neck, sighing with pleasure as you enjoy his scent. Tune in to how his hands feel on your skin. Slow down when kissing him, and notice all the sensations you experience. Enjoying these little moments is key to building intimacy.

Remember, he's not as picky as you think. I can pretty much guarantee that if your partner has a good libido, he is going to appreciate any gestures your inner vixen wants to make. Don't be scared to seduce him a little. Surprise him in the shower by jumping in and soaping him up, or cook a sensual dinner, clothes-free. His enthusiasm just might take your breath away.

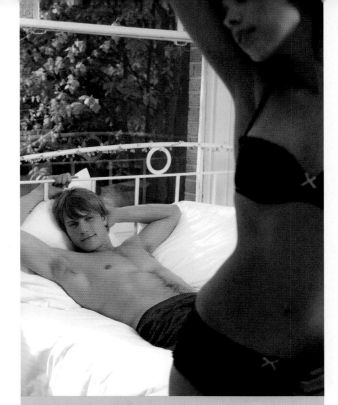

How to...

SEDUCE YOUR PARTNER

Once you dip your toe in the seduction pool, some of the intimidation factor will disappear. In fact, you will probably find that seduction is fun (it's meant to be)! If you still feel nervous about your role as seductress, talk to your partner or write him a note describing your intention to create more seduction in your lives.

1 Put on some sexy lingerie (if you feel anxious, see page 141 for more on body image in the bedroom).

2 Do a little striptease for him. Get yourself in the mood by lighting candles and turning on some music that gets you going. Then, take your clothing off piece by piece. It will feel more natural than you think.

3 Remember, confidence is key. If you must, "fake it 'til you make it"—and when you see how well he responds, you won't have to fake it for long!

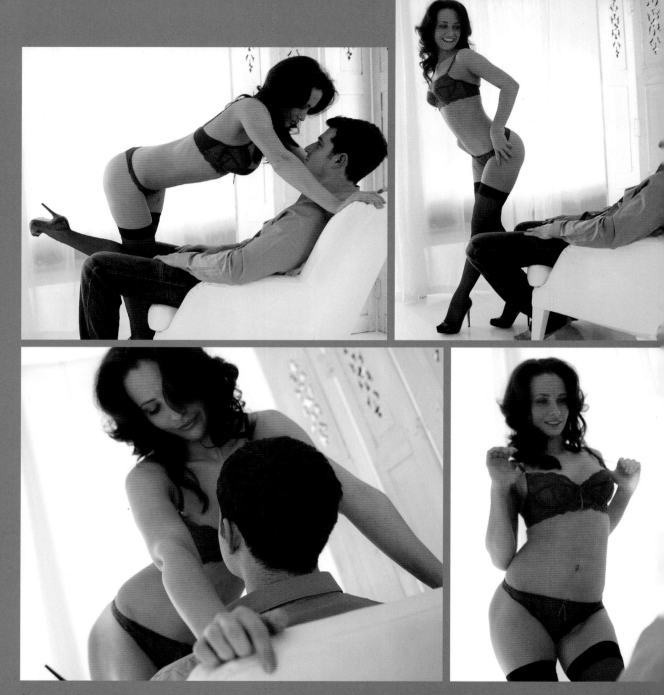

Lap dance
Vixens, it's time to sit your partner down for some serious seduction. Start with saucy lingerie and music that gets your blood pumping. Move slowly at first, building anticipation by brushing lightly against your partner, then stepping back so he can see you fully on display. Come closer as the layers come off, reveling in your vixen's power to allow him the touch he craves only when you feel the time is right.

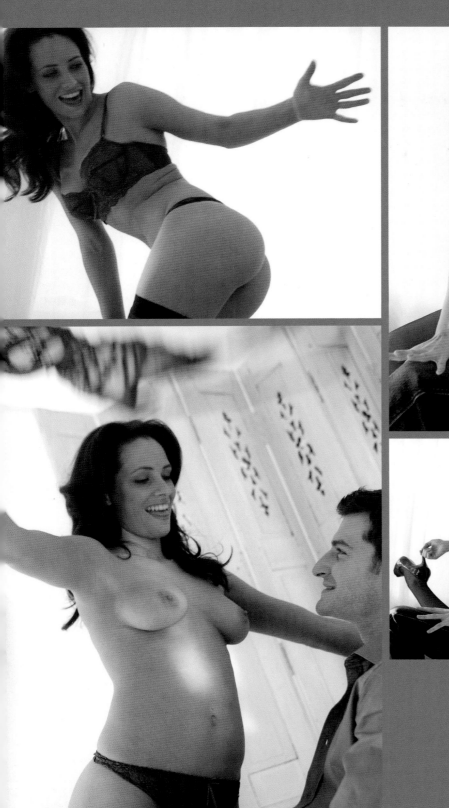
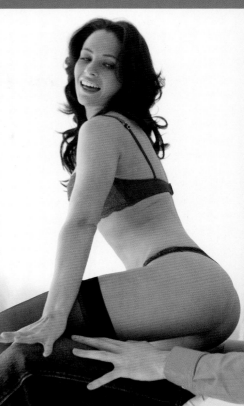
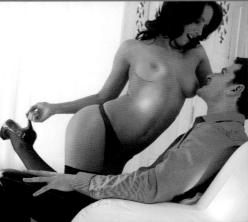

Making good sex great

By nature, humans are creatures of habit. We slip into routines and rely on old patterns to help guide us through life. This is easy, but it can threaten your sexual connection and spark. If you have been stuck in a relationship rut (however comfortable) for awhile, you may have a good sex life—but taking a step back to analyze your relationship and add a dose of adventure can transform your sex life into something truly great.

Getting out of a rut

It's easy to go to your favorite restaurant every date night. The maître d' knows you by name and you can always rely on the seafood risotto and the steak to be delicious. However, even an enjoyable rut is still a rut! In fact, it may be the worst kind, since it's hard to find the motivation to get out of it.

When your date night is about as exciting as watching paint dry, that lack of originality will impact sex after the date is over. In contrast, an exciting date can lead to a more spontaneous and adventurous experience in the bedroom later that night. So, make it a point to make some changes to your routine and do something adventurous together at least once or twice a month.

Change your schedule. For one month, commit to getting up at a certain time even on the weekends. Not only is this a good way to get your body into healthier sleep habits, but you might also be

The truth about...

CREATING SPACE IN YOUR RELATIONSHIP

To unleash your inner vixen, it's important to put away your need to control your partner. The more autonomy and respect you give him, the more love and affection he will funnel back to you. At the same time, you will be protecting the valuable masculine-feminine balance in your relationship. Great sex is a game of give-and-take, so improving your sex life isn't just about creating more sex appeal. It's also about allowing your partner more room to be the sexy man who stole your heart in the first place.

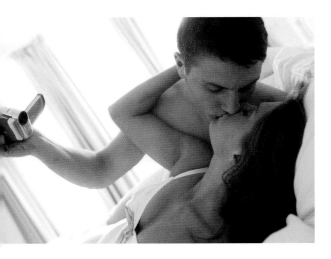

deserve sex, or you get so caught up in feelings of guilt that you don't have any energy left for sex. Try deciding that you will only be allowed to mentally beat yourself up while you are in the shower, or during 3–4 PM, or any other specific time. Then, promise yourself that you won't allow those thoughts to control your mind for the rest of the day.

Make use of the quickie. If you just don't have the oomph, remember that there is always the quickie. A quickie is better than nothing at all. It keeps a couple bonded, keeps their sexual response intact, and tides them over until they have the time and energy for a more extended sex session.

Making time for sex

When you're busy, it's important to schedule in time for sex. By doing this, you will allow yourself time to mentally wind down and prepare, along with some time to shave your legs and don some sexy lingerie. When you have more time during sex, you become more present, and can enjoy the experience a lot more. You can also take your time with foreplay and increase arousal levels for both of you.

If the idea of scheduling in sex doesn't sound romantic, consider the alternative: not having time for sex. That's the usual scenario for those with busy lives and lots of commitments. If you give scheduled sex a try, you'll find you can make it as sexy as spontaneous sex. In fact, you will probably start to look forward to it just as you look forward to any other date with your partner.

To build anticipation, try sending your partner a sexy email or text expressing how much you are thinking about your date. A note left near his bathroom sink can be effective, too, or you can slip it under his dinner plate if you are on a date. A bonus: Making gestures like these will encourage your partner to romance you in the same way.

surprised at how rising early can positively impact your life. Maybe you can fit in some early morning yoga, a good book, or a warm bath—or perhaps even a quickie! If you are struggling to find time to recharge and refresh, rising just a little earlier can be a good way to do this. When you challenge yourself to mix up your routine, you start to feel more successful, and your self-esteem and general happiness—both central to a great sex life—increase.

Have sex in one new place a month. Try sex in the car (not when you're driving, of course), sex on the kitchen countertop, sex in the shower—the possibilities are endless. Or, commit to trying one new sex position or technique each month, or to recording a steamy sex tape each month.

Stop feeling guilty. Women in particular often suffer from extreme feelings of guilt and regret (for more on this, see page 16). These feelings can kill your spirit and your libido. If you are carrying around pounds of emotional baggage, it's time to start letting it go, in the bedroom and beyond. This is especially true if you imagine that you don't

Rethinking your sexual expectations

Your expectations of your sex life, or sexpectations as I like to call them, can define your whole sexual experience. If you walk into the bedroom every night expecting to be ravaged just like the women in the romance novels you love, you will inevitably be let down when you discover your partner is already half asleep. Sex should be wonderful, bonding, and connecting, but it should also be real. Real love and sex might not have the same exaggerated appeal as what you see on television, but it has something much more valuable: the security that comes with fully knowing, understanding, and supporting another person, flaws and all.

Fictionalized romance

Ladies, put down the remote! Your addiction to romantic comedies might be harming your happiness in your real relationship. A recent study found that fans of romantic comedies are less likely to communicate with their partners and more likely to have unrealistic expectations of their sex lives and their relationships. The study, performed at Heriot-Watt University in Edinburgh, Scotland, interviewed students who had seen famous rom-com fare and found that they had a less realistic view of love.

Researchers theorize that this is because romantic comedies encourage us to believe in fate and destiny, rather than showing the inner workings of a strong relationship. Unlike real life, movies present love as something that happens overnight, lasts forever, and has only the most humorous of road bumps.

Real sex

Those of us who have been in a real-life relationship know that the reality is much different. The major thing that separates successful relationships from unsuccessful ones is how hard you are willing to work to maintain your connection. Of course, this hard work isn't always sexy. Nobody wants to watch Snow White and Prince Charming arguing in couples' therapy, or Jennifer Lopez and Matthew McConaughey having a dry spell in the bedroom. Yet this is the reality of what goes on inside the homes and hearts of lovers everywhere.

Unfortunately, our patience and commitment might be even more strained if we have unrealistic expectations, specifically for our sex lives. Not only do romantic comedies not show the day-to-day effort that goes into real relationships, they also don't show the effort that goes into real sex lives. Real sex isn't always spontaneous, nor is it always orgasmic, and most couples have to work to keep sex special. Everyone's sex life has ebbs and flows, and there are times when we all feel tired, stressed, and downright uninterested. Of course, you can change things you dislike about your sex life, but don't expect changes to happen overnight or for your relationship to then be perfect. Sometimes all you will have the energy for is what I call "maintenance sex"—routine, quick, and to-the-point. That's okay, as long as you plan for fireworks sometime in the near future.

Saying yes to sex

Still, there will always be times when you aren't in the mood for sex. In my experience, however, I find that women too quickly reject their partners. On the one hand, you should never do anything sexually that makes you uncomfortable. On the other hand, you shouldn't reject your partner outright all the time.

Shutting down your partner every night simply isn't fair to him. The two of you have agreed to be each other's sexual outlet, and if he isn't getting what he needs from you, it can dramatically affect his mood and your relationship (for more on this, see page 181).

A good rule of thumb is this: Have sex whenever your partner asks, and vice versa. As long as the amount of sex that your partner asks for is not exorbitant, try considering sex even when you aren't in the mood. Aside from making your partner happy, you will benefit from his increased connection. Men feel emotionally connected when they have sex, and women want sex when they feel emotionally connected. So, the more you have sex, the more connected your partner will feel and act, which in turn will increase your sexual desire—a win-win situation if ever there was one.

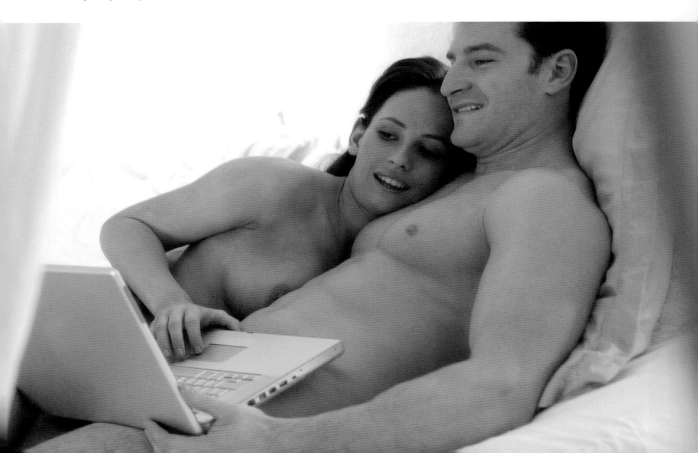

Orgasm

Unfortunately, there are a lot of unrealistic expectations around sex. One of these is that intercourse should bring easy orgasm for both men and women. This is simply not true. Men and women's bodies reach orgasm in different ways, and understanding this is key in ensuring that you both achieve the ultimate climax of sexual pleasure.

The anatomy of orgasm

To start with, let me just remind you that only one-third of women can reach an orgasm during intercourse. I've found that most women are surprised by this statistic, in addition to feeling incredibly relieved. In fact, knowing this can be half the battle, since a big part of having an orgasm is getting over the pressure to have one. If you become frustrated with your orgasmic abilities, remember this: Most women cannot reach orgasm during intercourse without learning some specific techniques to make it happen.

A simple anatomy lesson is the first step. While many women love the sensation of penetration and the feeling of closeness it allows with their partner, it is not the magical path to orgasm that movies and popular media have made it seem. For two-thirds of women at least, a little more legwork is needed. The real magic button for women is the clitoris, and this is the area you probably need to pay more attention to with your partner. It will usually be up to you to give him some gentle guidance. Done right, it will be satisfying for him to please you in the way you want to be pleased.

Slowing sex down

But first, back to what I said earlier. The surest way not to have an orgasm is to focus on it incessantly. Instead, relax and let sensations envelop you. Exist in your body instead of in your head, making an effort to forget about other worries or distractions. Let your partner know that your orgasm is something that will come with time, so to speak, and in the meantime, see where sex takes you. Try kissing and touching until you get really aroused, then pulling back a bit. In addition to giving you enough time to get fully aroused, this will help your partner stay in the game longer, which most women need to ultimately make it to orgasm.

Techniques for orgasm

Now, the big question is, how do you incorporate the right techniques and teach your partner about what brings you to a point of climax in a way that doesn't feel like rejection? The answer is two-pronged: self-stimulation and communication. You may already be a step ahead in that you masturbate and know how to bring yourself to orgasm. Good for you! I tell women everyday that self-stimulation is the best way to figure out what works for them.

What you need to do now is pay closer attention to what you are doing when you masturbate. Which parts do you touch, what rhythm do you use, what other erogenous zones are especially sensitive for you? Next, put these observations to work during sex with your partner. One way to do this is to voice suggestions as positive affirmation, such as "It turns me on when you touch me there," or "I love it when you stroke me there a little harder." You can also show your partner what you want by demonstrating through self-stimulation in front of him, and even describing the sensation.

If these options seem too daunting, use nonverbal cues instead. Take his hand and put it where you want him to touch. Moan, stroke, or kiss him when he does something you like. A little verbal reinforcement can work, too, such as "oh yeah!" or "right there!" All of these clues will help him understand what you like—and with a little practice, he will start to learn what pleases you and you will do less directing.

Another way to increase your chances of orgasm is to try positions that stimulate the clitoris. Woman-on-top positions often provide more clitoral stimulation than man-on-top, and also allow you to direct the speed and rhythm. You can also use your hand or a small vibrator to stimulate your clitoris during penetration, or ask your partner to do this for you (for more on sex toys, see pages 166–167).

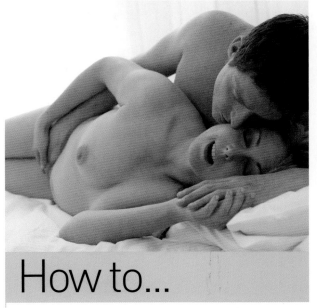

How to...

SELF-STIMULATE IN FRONT OF YOUR PARTNER

Most men find the thought of women enjoying self-stimulation highly erotic. When you pleasure yourself in front of him, he sees you as comfortable with your body, desirous of him, and passionate—all positives. He will likely love it, but it may be harder for you. Here's a good way to go about it.

1 Ask your partner if he has ever thought about you touching yourself, or if he has ever fantasized about doing so in front of you.

2 Or, start off by touching your self and your genitals during sexual play. Then, try doing this while you are kissing or pressed close to each other.

3 If you still feel self-conscious, ask your partner to share the experience by self-stimulating with you.

Positions with a purpose

New positions can open you up to different kinds of penetration and stimulation, and experimenting with them is an easy way to bring more fun and spontaneity into the bedroom—it literally forces you to look at things from a different point of view. Not to mention, you can use different positions to work toward relationship goals, whether you want to feel more connected, be more spontaneous, or regain intimacy after a fight.

Exploring your options

Not every position is going to work for you and your partner. In fact, some positions might even make you laugh more than they turn you on! That's half the fun of experimenting. Of course, the other half of the fun is discovering an amazing new position that you hadn't been bold enough to try before.

Regardless of which position you are trying out, keep in mind that lubrication is an important component. Certain positions lend themselves to deeper or tighter penetration, which can be painful at first if you don't apply a generous amount of lubrication. You should also talk to your partner if you encounter a position that simply doesn't work for you, or if you find an angle to be uncomfortable.

The right pillow can be equally revolutionary. This great bedroom accessory can completely revamp a position or add a new twist to an old favorite. (For example, try placing a pillow under your hips during the missionary position, which can intensify penetration and improve your angle for orgasm.) You might also find that some positions are better equipped for the floor (especially if you have a particularly high mattress), in which case pillows are a great tool for making the floor more sensual, comfortable, and inviting. If you have knee or back problems, pillows can also be a good way to provide support and reduce joint strain during sex. Finding the little tricks that work for you is what makes your own sex life intimately yours.

The intimacy builder (right) Sometimes sex
doesn't need any bells or whistles. When what you want is intimacy and connection, lie on your sides and face each other. Wrap your legs around each other, with your top leg wrapped around his back, and his top leg bent over your lower leg. This is a very intimate position that will bond you and heighten your arousal.

Sideways sex

There's something gentle and loving about sex from the side, where both partners are on equal ground and can caress and stroke to their heart's content. Perhaps this is why the Kama Sutra says sideways sex is perfect for new lovers. New or old, practice these positions whenever you want real closeness.

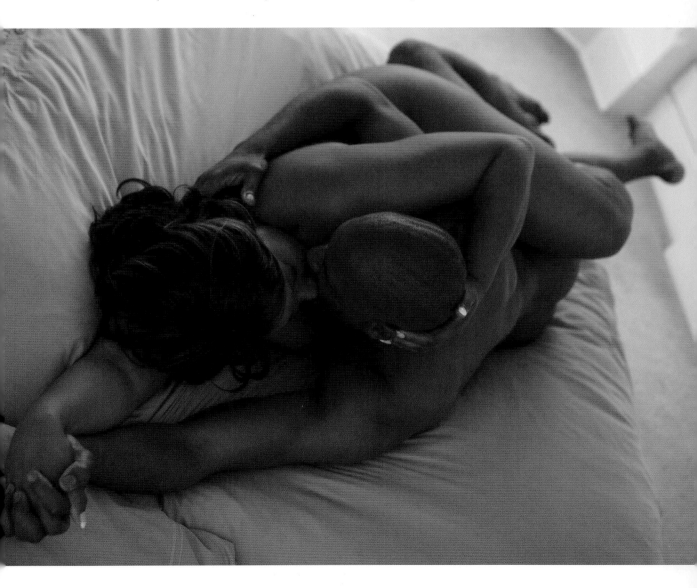

Tender lovemaking

Nothing can rival the deep intimacy that sex this close can bring. Face-to-face, arms and legs entwined, lovemaking like this is healing in its slow, sultry passion. It's the perfect way to reconnect after you've spent time apart or had an argument. Switching the position away from the traditional missionary can make things a bit more exciting, and will help ensure that you receive the type of clitoral stimulation you need.

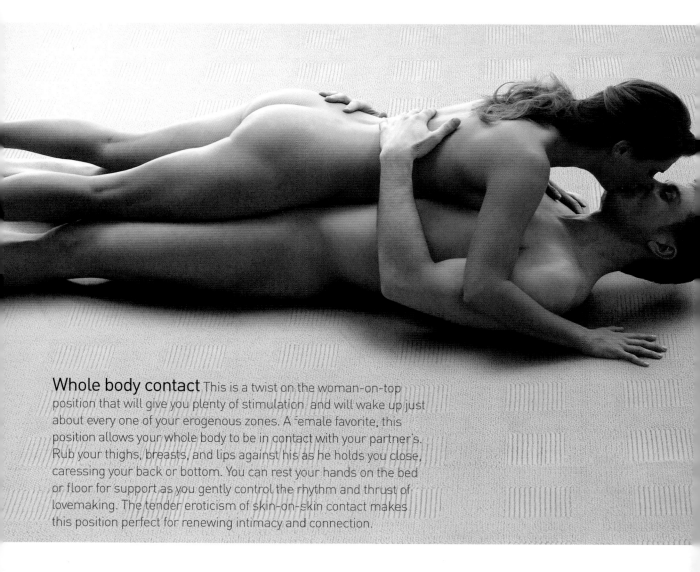

Whole body contact This is a twist on the woman-on-top position that will give you plenty of stimulation, and will wake up just about every one of your erogenous zones. A female favorite, this position allows your whole body to be in contact with your partner's. Rub your thighs, breasts, and lips against his as he holds you close, caressing your back or bottom. You can rest your hands on the bed or floor for support as you gently control the rhythm and thrust of lovemaking. The tender eroticism of skin-on-skin contact makes this position perfect for renewing intimacy and connection.

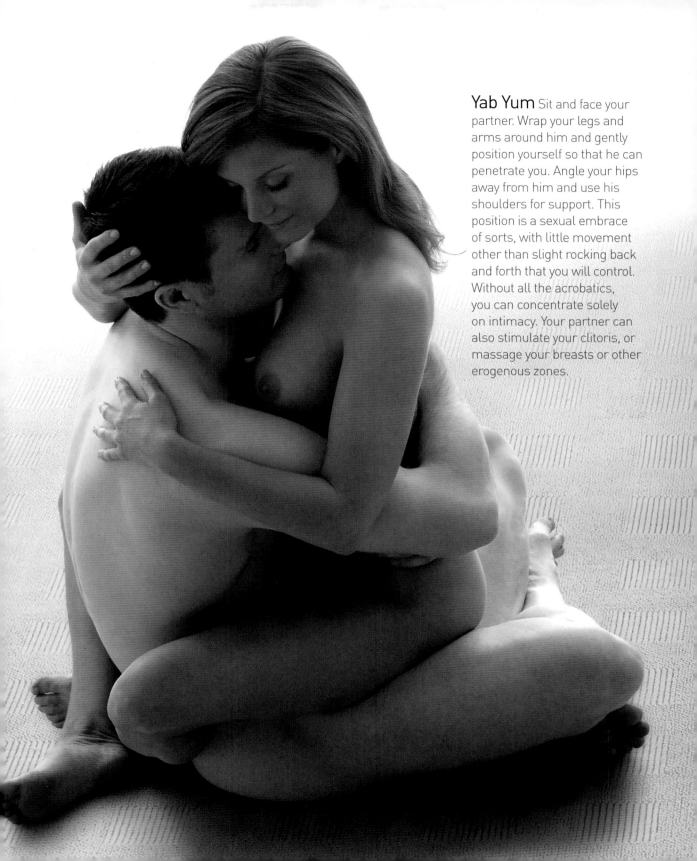

Yab Yum Sit and face your partner. Wrap your legs and arms around him and gently position yourself so that he can penetrate you. Angle your hips away from him and use his shoulders for support. This position is a sexual embrace of sorts, with little movement other than slight rocking back and forth that you will control. Without all the acrobatics, you can concentrate solely on intimacy. Your partner can also stimulate your clitoris, or massage your breasts or other erogenous zones.

The right penetration

Make some very small changes to the classic lovemaking positions and you will probably find that your orgasmic ability expands immeasurably. Remember, it's all about clitoral stimulation. Slowing down stimulation, making sure that your partner is positioned to hit just the right spot, and adding in a few new props are key to your climax.

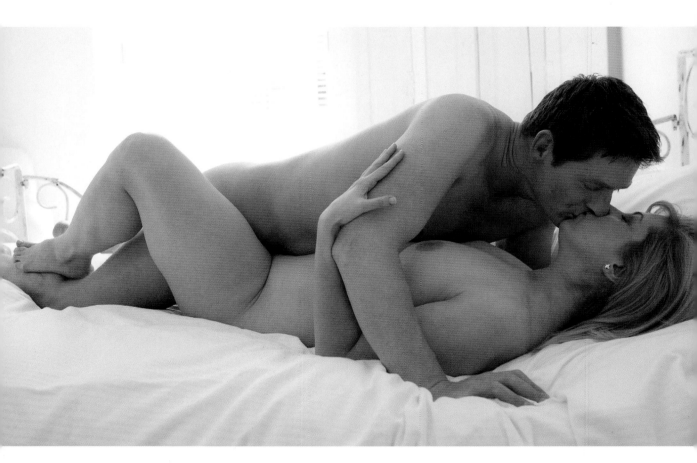

The orgasm enhancer CAT, or Coital Alignment Technique, is a twist on the traditional missionary position—and well-loved by women everywhere! With your partner on top, he lifts his hips up and over your hips, and then gently rocks back and forth. The base of his pelvic bone should fit against your clitoris, which lets him thrust deeply while maximizing clitoral stimulation for you. This position is also great for G-spot stimulation because it gives you lots of friction.

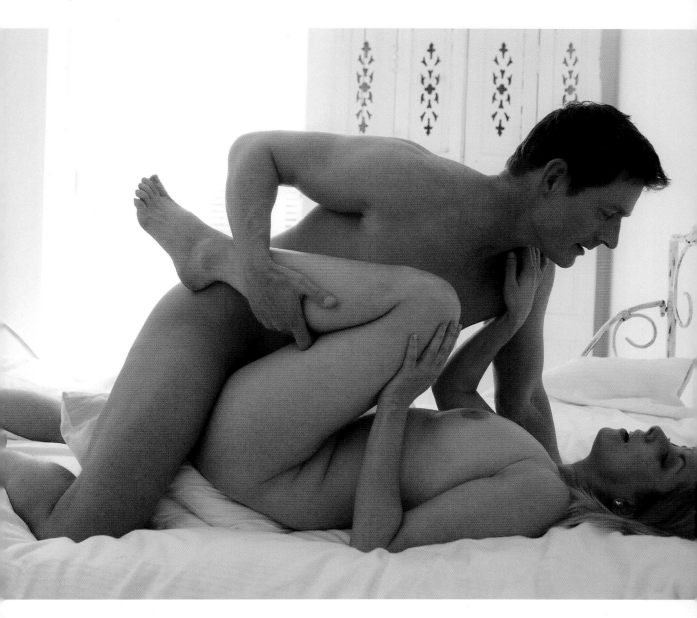

The new classic For nights when you are tired but want to feel close, stick with what's comfortable and up your pleasure quotient with some well-placed props. Pillows are an essential bedroom tool, and can add a new twist to a favorite position. Here's what to do: Place a pillow under your hips so that your hips are at a slightly higher angle. Your partner can then enter you at a deeper and more erotic angle, for the type of penetration that is perfect for both of you.

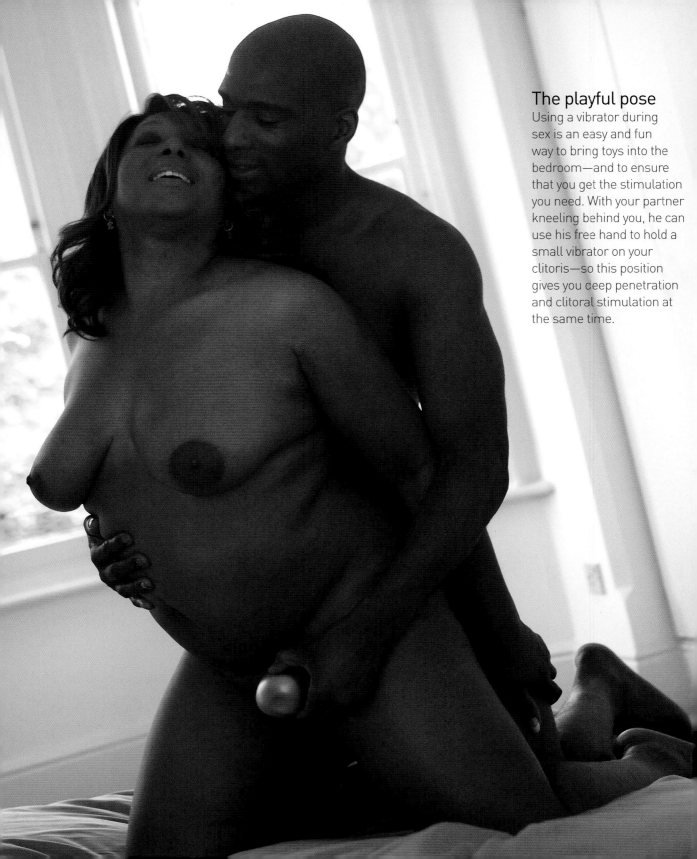

The playful pose

Using a vibrator during sex is an easy and fun way to bring toys into the bedroom—and to ensure that you get the stimulation you need. With your partner kneeling behind you, he can use his free hand to hold a small vibrator on your clitoris—so this position gives you deep penetration and clitoral stimulation at the same time.

Targeted touch

Toys can truly revolutionize your bedroom experience. Aside from the excitement that comes from their added dose of naughtiness, the right toy can increase stimulation and make all those positions your partner loves equally satisfying for you. If you're not quite ready to bring any type of prop into the bedroom, manual touch can have the same erotic effect.

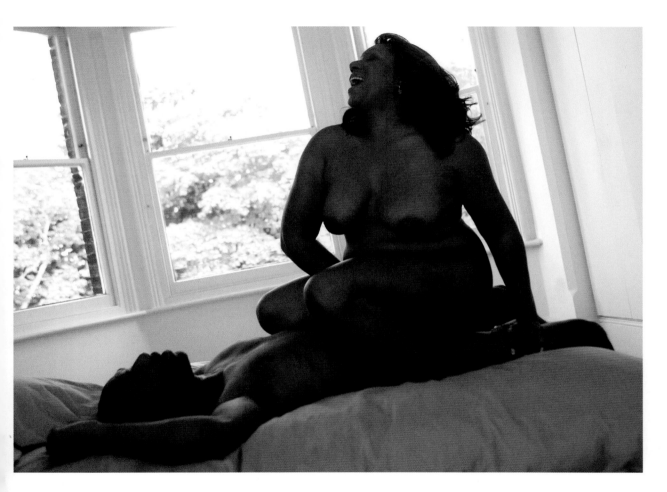

The stimulation booster Woman-on-top positions help ensure that you get the stimulation you need, and are also thrillingly erotic for your partner. Try this sometime when you are both looking for a little bit of adventure. To start, take control by straddling him. He will get a view of your assets, while you can manually stimulate your clitoris. Being in command also allows you to decide the rhythm and depth of penetration.

Pure seduction

One of the best ways to express your needs in the bedroom is to simply show your partner what you want. Taking charge in this way not only allows you to stay in control of the pace and depth of penetration, it is also a huge turn-on for your partner. Remember, men like to be pursued occasionally. So, show him that you want him—and get what you want in the process.

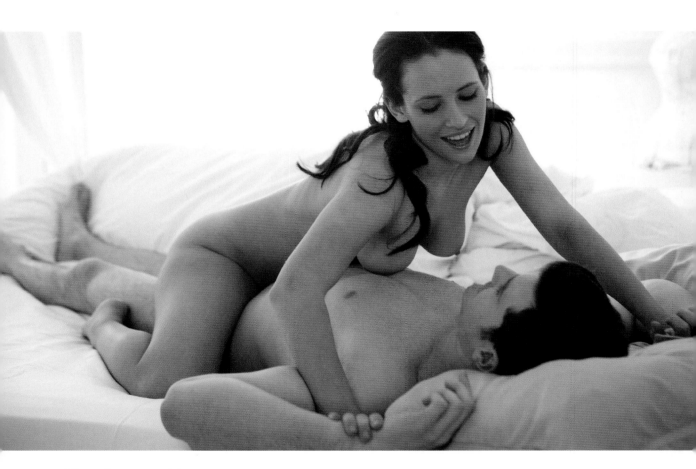

The vixen position Taking charge in the bedroom is easier than you might think! In fact, once you see how fun, not to mention pleasurable, it can be, it will revolutionize the way you think about sex. A bonus? Seeing you as the initiator will be a huge turn-on for him. To start, try straddling your partner and playfully pinning him down as you thrust together at varying levels of penetration. Enjoy the natural friction this move creates—as well as the opportunity to tap into your inner vixen and take charge of your sexual pleasure.

Around the house

Sex outside the bedroom can make quick lovemaking sessions even more thrilling and instantly gratifying. Try the stairs, the kitchen counter, that huge arm chair in the living room, or anywhere else that strikes your fancy and allows for a daring-yet-discreet display of passion.

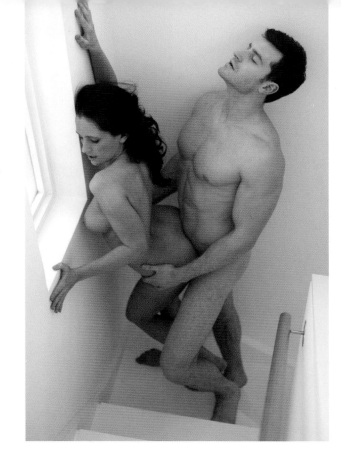

The can't-wait-to-get-upstairs move

Next time you come home with your heart racing from a hot date, try this for instant satisfaction: Rest on the stairs while he enters you from on top, or use the rails to prop up your leg or give yourself leverage. You can also do man-from-behind on the stairs, with both of you standing, him one step down from you.

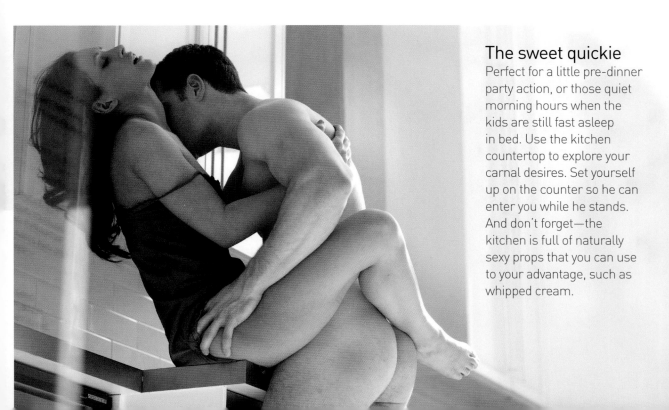

The sweet quickie

Perfect for a little pre-dinner party action, or those quiet morning hours when the kids are still fast asleep in bed. Use the kitchen countertop to explore your carnal desires. Set yourself up on the counter so he can enter you while he stands. And don't forget—the kitchen is full of naturally sexy props that you can use to your advantage, such as whipped cream.

Wet sex

There's something about sex under water—that slippery, sultry sensation offers a special kind of sensual thrill. Seek out alone time in the bath or shower to take full advantage of the naturally sexy scenarios that present themselves every day. Positions like these are perfect for pre-work sex on a weekday morning, or to give a joint workout session a steamy ending.

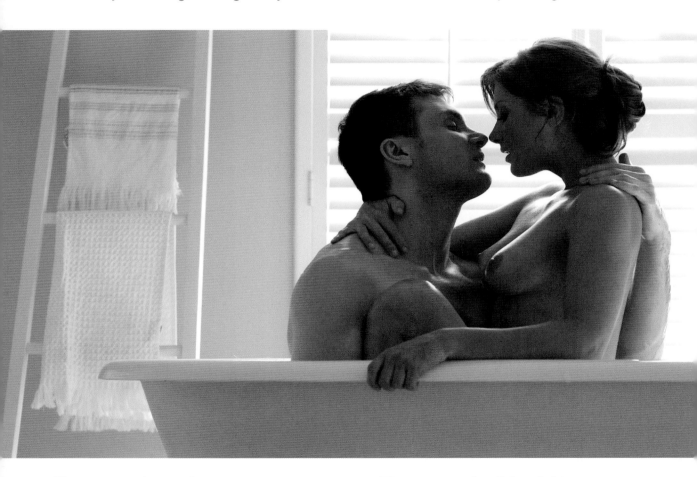

The romantic rendezvous (above) The next time you want passion, look just a little beyond the bedroom. The bathtub is a great place for romance, especially if you set the scene with a few bubbles and candles. While your partner kneels, gently kneel over him and rock back and forth. Use a hand to stimulate your clitoris as you slip and slide back and forth.

The wet-and-wild quickie (right) Showering together will make your everyday routine a lot sexier. It adds a sense of spontaneity to sex, and is also a great place to explore because everything is slippery and sensual. One of the best shower-time positions is this: bend slightly at the waist while your partner enters you, using the wall to maintain your balance.

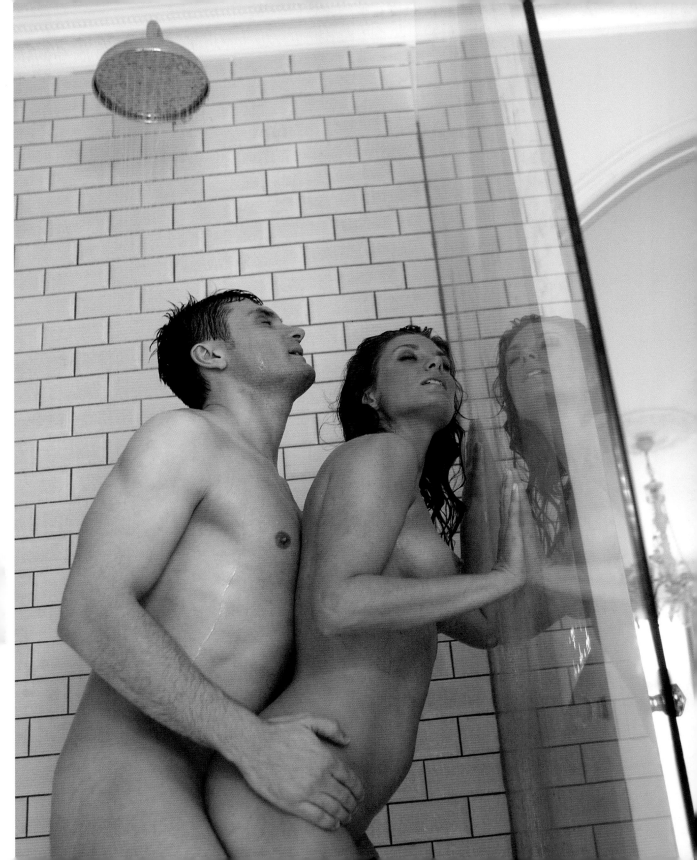

Sex toys

Sex toys are an essential part of the vixen tool kit. Not only can they increase arousal and add spice to your sex life, they can also teach you more about your own personal sexual response. Familiarize yourself with the many options available, and make a promise to your partner and yourself that you'll add one or two toys into your intimacy mix.

Vibrators

If you are like most people, you probably think "vibrators" when you think sex toys. The vibrator is the classic toy for women, used to increase pleasure and clitoral stimulation during sex, or during self-stimulation. Every year more and more types become available, so there truly is an option for every woman. If the thought of shopping for sex toys in person makes you nervous, erotica websites make this process easy. Simply browse online, then have a discreet package delivered to your door.

Now, let's go over the options. The classic external vibrator allows for direct clitoral stimulation, and can be placed on the vulva or other erogenous zones. Other toys are penis-shaped (some more abstract than others) for penetration, and there are some that also vibrate. Other vibrators come with attachments that you insert into the vagina while the outer piece vibrates against your clitoris. Take some time to experiment with a few of these options, and find the stimulation that works for you It should be a fun journey, and you will no doubt end with a few favorites.

G-spot stimulators

You may never have encountered your G-spot before—in fact, many women think this is a myth! If you fall in this category, consider a vibrator that was designed for the sole purpose of helping you find this female erogenous zone. (See diagram on page 106 for more on the location of the G-spot.) G-spot stimulators can help you locate this hot spot quickly and easily, taking away any guesswork or fruitless searching on your part.

Different designs and levels of intensity mean that you can choose a toy that's perfect for your needs. Most G-spot stimulators are penis-shaped, but curved at the end to give you easy and direct access to this hot spot. Some also vibrate for added

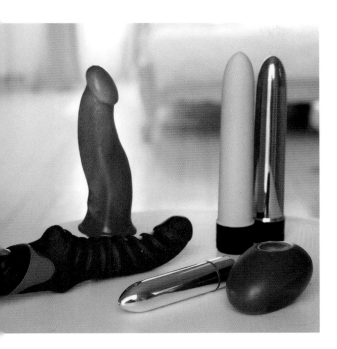

Flavored lubricants Flavored lubricants are a fun, sexy way to spice up your oral sex adventures. From cherry to pina colada to chocolate to vanilla, there is a flavor for everyone! Experiment until you find your favorites.

Durex Play Utopia This enhancement gel, created by the famous condom company, increases arousal in women by bringing more intense sensations to erogenous zones like the clitoris. Utopia contains an ingredient called L-Arginine, which is an amino acid that relaxes muscles around blood vessels to increase blood flow to the female genitals. Utopia also contains propylene glycol, which creates a warming sensation that can increase your sexual response. You can try applying Utopia on your clitoris and the rest of your genitals before sex in order to maximize sensation and arousal.

Zestra This all-natural botanical oil is applied to the genitals before foreplay, and works to create a tingling sensation and increased arousal. In clinical trials, Zestra was proven to enhance sexual desire, arousal, and orgasmic ability. Some women who use Zestra report that their partner experiences increased sexual arousal as well, although it is unclear whether this is due to their excitement at their partner's arousal or their own increased desire.

sensation and intensity. Even if you are already well versed in your G-spot, these toys can help you discover different kinds of stimulation and experience more intense G-spot orgasms. Some combine G-spot and clitoral vibratory stimulation in one, for the ultimate blended orgasm.

Spicing things up

Beyond vibrators and G-spot stimulators, there is a whole world of erotic tools out there! If you are looking for more fun ways to spice up your sex life, consider these out-of-the-box erotic treats:

Vibrating panties These panties include a small clitoral simulator that can be operated by a remote, allowing your partner to stimulate you without using his hands. For the truly daring, try wearing a pair of these panties to a party and having your partner stimulate you from up to 12 feet away!

66 Different levels of intensity mean that you can choose a toy that's perfect for your needs. 99

Fantasy

Fantasy is an important part of your sexuality. The erotic images and ideas that you dream up are what fuel your sexuality and keep you in touch with your desires. The more you can connect with an internal sexual fantasy life, the more your inner vixen thrives, and the better your sex life will be.

Everyday fantasy

It might sound strange, but it's true—fantasy can be a part of your daily routine. In fact, it should be and here's why: The more you fantasize and think about sex, the easier it will be for you to switch into naughty mode with your partner. Fantasy is really the only time when you can be in complete control of your sexual circumstances, and it can inspire a much greater sexual connection when you actually are in the moment. An active fantasy life helps you learn about what turns you on and helps you experience more satisfaction in the bedroom.

If you find yourself feeling guilty or even a bit embarrassed about your fantasies, just remind yourself: Fantasy isn't reality. It doesn't hurt anyone, including your partner (who likely has a few zillion fantasies himself!). Whether you are dreaming about a Hollywood celeb, a real-life crush, or your partner, fantasy is a fun and safe way to explore your desires.

Remember, too, that just because you fantasize about hooking up with a sexy stranger doesn't mean that you actually want to cheat on your partner. Nor does fantasizing about taking part in a threesome or playing submission and domination games mean that you actually want to try those things in real life. Most fantasies are just that— fantasies. You don't have to take them any further unless you choose to, so there is no need to put any limits or shame on your mental playground.

Fantasy for beginners

If you are new to the world of fantasy, don't worry. It is easy to become immersed in your own fantasy land, even if you haven't done it before. To start, try drawing inspiration from movies, books, art, or even music—whatever is sensual to you (for resources that can help, see page 251). The world is a very erotic place, all you have to do is tap into that energy!

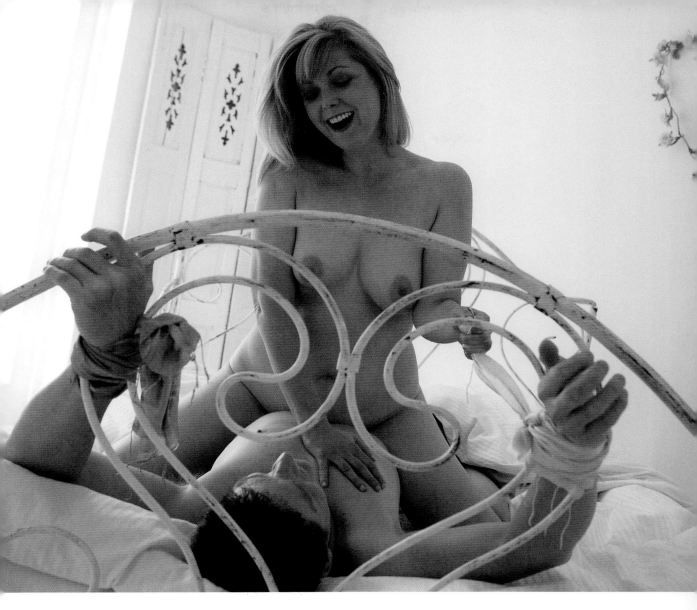

Next, spend some time by yourself thinking about different erotic scenarios. Try to discover what is so sexy to you about those particular situations. Is it that you are completely in control? Is it that you feel like your partner can't wait to have you? Once you discover what really turns you on, playing out your fantasies in real life will become much easier. For example, if you know that the thought of your partner having to have you *right now* turns you on, explore that by having sex somewhere a little bit

dangerous, such as in the restroom at a party or in the backseat of your car. If you want to be in control, play out a policewoman fantasy and pull your partner over for a ticket, or be the sexy teacher with the innocent student. (Remember, it's fantasy, so even if it is illegal and completely inappropriate in real life, in your imagination it's all okay.) Other power role-play fantasies people often enjoy are doctor/patient, boss/employee, sexy stranger you meet randomly—the sky is truly the limit!

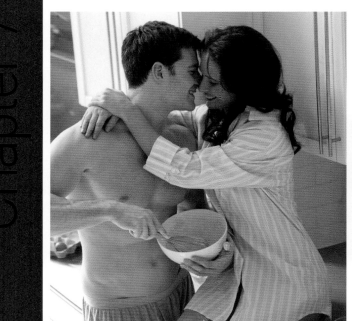

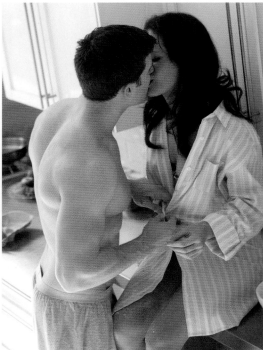

Chapter 7

Making your relationship matter

There is no denying the fact that every strong partnership is based on strong communication. Understanding how your partner communicates, and conveying your own needs, are the keys that can unlock a lifetime of support and love. To do this, you must commit to fighting fairly, seeking out compromise, prioritizing intimacy, and choosing each other's happiness first and foremost.

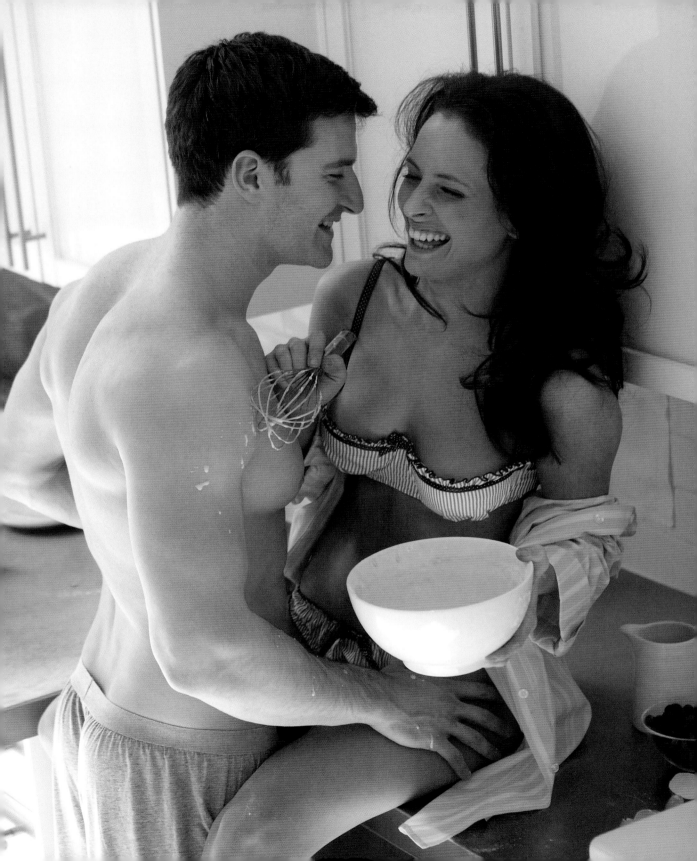

It's common knowledge that good communication is one of the keys to a happy relationship. So, it's no surprise that examining the way you communicate with your partner is an important step toward making your relationship the best it can be. Think about the questions below, notice what habits might contribute to miscommunication or conflict, and then read on to learn how to replace those habits with the healthy communication tools that are the foundation for a lifetime of relationship happiness.

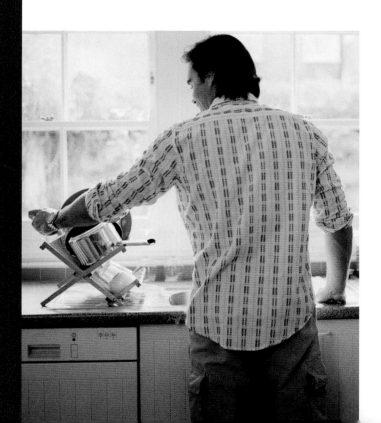

1 YOUR PARTNER PROMISES TO HELP YOU CLEAN THE

house prior to having his friends over. However, when the time rolls around, he is zoned out in front of the computer and seems deaf to the sounds of vacuuming around him. You:

A Slam down the vacuum and leave the house without saying a word. If he isn't going to help, then he can entertain his friends on his own.

B Finish the cleaning on your own and sit tight-lipped and silent throughout his friends' visit. It's not your fault that you are in a bad mood—maybe he will actually help you next time you have guests!

C Ask him plainly and politely to fulfill his promise to help you, by saying something such as, "Your friends will be here in an hour. If I vacuum and dust, can you take out the trash and handle the dishes?"

2 YOUR PARTNER HAS BEEN WORKING LATE A LOT.

Although you are starting to feel neglected and lonely, you have tried not to complain. However, when he completely forgets about your Saturday date night, you:

A Get into a screaming match with him when he gets home from work. He needs to know that you won't be mistreated like this.

B Give him the cold shoulder, but act like nothing is wrong. Then, when your next date night comes around, you purposefully make other plans.

C Sit down with him and explain that your feelings are hurt by saying, "When you forget our date night, I feel sad because it makes me think that I am not important to you and that you would rather work than spend time alone with me."

3 YOU HAVE A RARE DINNER OUT SCHEDULED WITH

your girlfriends. You ask your husband to make sure your son is in bed by 8 PM. However, when you return home at 10 PM, you discover that he is still awake and watching TV in bed with your husband. You:

Ⓐ Sigh and say, "I knew I couldn't trust you to be responsible for his bedtime," then send your kid to bed.

Ⓑ Ask your son to go to bed and then call your sister to complain about your lazy and irresponsible husband.

Ⓒ Lie down next to them and enjoy some downtime with your favorite men for a few minutes, then get up and put your son to bed together.

4 YOU RECENTLY JOINED FACEBOOK AND HAVE BEEN SPENDING A LOT OF TIME

reconnecting with old friends online. However, when your husband finds out that one of these old friends is actually an ex-boyfriend of yours, he gets very upset and demands that you close your account. You:

Ⓐ Refuse to give in and say, "I can't help it if you have a jealousy problem.

Be as paranoid as you want. I am not doing anything wrong, so there is no reason for you to be jealous."

Ⓑ Pretend to close your account but keep it open and log in when he isn't around. You don't have anything to hide, but you don't want to argue about it.

Ⓒ Talk to him about why this makes him uncomfortable and try to come to a compromise, perhaps by refraining from communicating with your ex or even "defriending" him. At the end of the day, it's more important to keep the peace with your husband than to keep in contact with someone who is a virtual stranger to you now.

5 YOUR PARTNER HAS BEEN OFFERED A NEW JOB

that allows him plenty of opportunity for upward growth. For the first time in years, he is excited about his career and his professional future. However, it requires more travel and doesn't pay as much as his current job. When he asks you for your opinion, you say:

Ⓐ "I don't think we should be taking a pay cut right now. Maybe in a few years when the kids are done with school."

Ⓑ "What's most important is that you are happy. The kids and I will be fine. Don't worry about us!"

Ⓒ "Congratulations! Let's talk about the ways we can manage with less money and more travel, so the kids and I don't miss you too much."

A-type answers show that you are fighting to win. You think that by yelling the loudest or being the toughest, you can win every argument and bully your partner into submission. This isn't the way to create healthy communication, however, and it will negatively impact your relationship happiness and security in the long run.

B-type answers indicate that you avoid confrontation and tend to show your anger through passive-aggressive actions. Instead of sharing your true feelings, you express your hurt by holding onto your anger for days—or even weeks—and shutting out your partner. This makes it very hard for him to know what you need to be happy in your relationship.

C-type answers mean that you are able to be flexible, and are more confident in expressing your needs to your partner and hearing his needs in return. Congratulations! Responding in this way means that you are fighting to love, not to win (for more on this, see page 176).

❝Examining how you communicate will help you make your relationship the best it can be.❞

The modern relationship

Gender roles have changed dramatically over the last 20 years, and as a result, the way men and women relate to one another has also evolved. Today's women are empowered more than ever before—sexually, in relationships, and in every other part of life. We can pursue any field we desire, have a family, start a business, and accomplish pretty much any other goal we set. And yet, these accomplishments have in a sense become a new obstacle. Our very busyness prevents us from creating the relationships we truly want.

Evolving sexual relationships

One of the biggest areas in which relationships have changed in recent years is in the bedroom. In the past, we believed the messages we were told: that only "bad girls" enjoy sex and ask for what they want. "Nice girls," on the other hand, were supposed to meet the needs of their partners, but not be too assertive in the bedroom. Because of this, women often did not seek their own orgasms or try to improve their sex lives. In addition, women rarely talked about their sex lives with anyone, even their own doctors. All of this shame and silence led to numerous problems in the bedroom.

With the modern age and their newfound power, women have redefined themselves as individuals and as partners. We no longer believe that our role is in the home unless we want it to be. We also no longer subscribe to the notion that sex is something that only men enjoy. Thankfully, most women now know that sexual desire is an important part of who we are as human beings, and that sexual satisfaction is central to relationship satisfaction. In short, we aren't ashamed about sex any more. Women now feel more comfortable than ever making their sexual needs a priority, and talking about their sexuality with their partners and their doctors. In addition to strengthening the trust and equality in relationships, this means that women are now able to take charge of their reproductive health and determine when (or if) they want to have children.

The relationship forecast

However, we still haven't reached relationship utopia. Although women can now apparently have it all, this new juggling act of roles comes with a hefty price tag. We now know that we can build and enjoy an equal and fulfilling relationship, but we are often so busy and stressed that we don't have the time or energy to do so. This is because

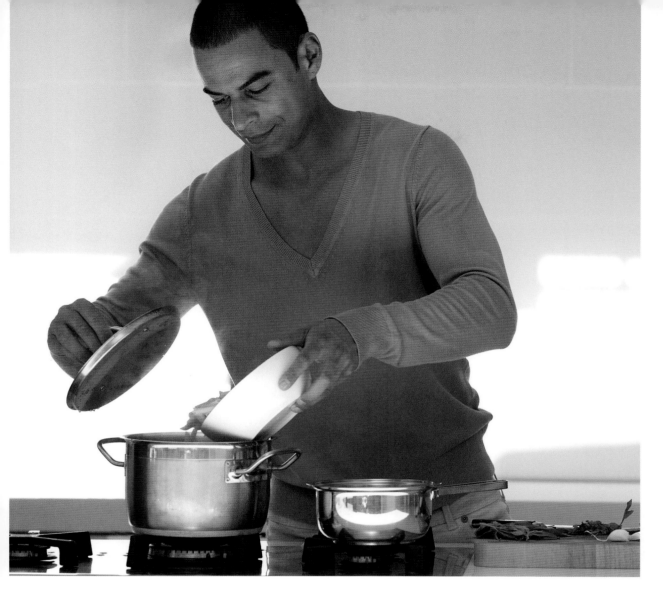

having too much on the to-do list separates us from identifying our needs and protecting our happiness. It is the dilemma of the modern relationship: how to fulfill your personal ambitions and realize that your own relationship satisfaction—including your sex life—must be a priority in order for it to succeed.

Modern love means that we are equal to our partner in work, life, love, child rearing, and sexual satisfaction. Couples today are getting there. However, women still undertake the majority of parenting and household responsibilities. This is something that needs to change as we move into a modern frontier and build the happy, fulfilling relationships we all want. Men now need to truly be partners in every sense of the word, whether that means putting the kids to bed, vacuuming the carpets, or other activities previously thought to be in the female domain. Women need to let their partners help them in this way, and relinquish the idea that only they can do it "right." To live in a place of modern love is the goal of every relationship. To get there, you simply need the right tools and the right mindset.

Fighting to love

Arguments are an inevitable part of any relationship. They are even healthy for your relationship if done well. No matter how happy you are, there will always be issues on which you and your partner don't see eye to eye. Addressing these issues, rather than ignoring them or pretending they don't exist, is a crucial part of developing and maintaining a healthy relationship.

The right way to fight

The difference between fighting to love and fighting to win is pretty simple. When you fight to win, you are putting your need to be right above your partner's feelings and your relationship. When you fight to love, you aren't fighting for yourself or fighting to be right. You are fighting for your relationship, and for positive changes that will grow your connection and your bond. The truth is that the momentary sense of safety or feeling of vindication that you get when you are "right," or when you badger your partner into an apology, pales in comparison to the feeling you get when your relationship is stable and your communication is healthy.

Yet, however simple the idea of fighting to love is, it isn't always easy in practice. Many of us learned poor communication patterns from our parents' way of fighting, and unlearning these lessons can be difficult, particularly if they are already established within our relationship. Creating strong communication patterns isn't always easy, but it is the best thing you can do for your mental health and your relationship.

Changing your routine

Many couples consider their communication style to be "normal," and therefore healthy—or at least not unhealthy. You know in theory that you shouldn't engage in a screaming match with your partner, or slam doors or insult each other. However, if that's what you saw growing up, and that's the way you have always communicated, you might consider it par for the course. After all, you might reason, no one has a completely harmonious relationship. Everyone loses their temper from time to time.

While it is true that no relationship is perfect and that every couple argues, ignoring or rationalizing constant bickering and anger can cause serious problems in your relationship. Every time you cross that line and begin communicating in an unhealthy, destructive, or downright vicious way, you erode your bond and decrease the feeling of safety and trust in your relationship.

So, make a commitment to fight for the relationship, not just for yourself. To start taking responsibility for your role, share this commitment verbally with your partner. Say something like, "I know that we are fighting a lot, and that I'm not doing my part to argue with you in a loving and constructive way. I am making a commitment to change that, and I won't allow myself to get carried away by anger or the need to be right." You don't need to ask your partner to commit to this as well. It's likely that he will choose to make a similar verbal commitment, but even if he doesn't, you will change the fighting dynamics simply by shifting your own attitude and approach.

> **❝ Creating strong communication patterns is the best thing you can do for your relationship. ❞**

Taking responsibility

As we discussed in Chapter 1, taking responsibility is the only way to communicate well and to build a happy relationship. If you blame your partner for your relationship issues, you are not only being unfair, you are preventing yourself from experiencing peace in this very important part of your life.

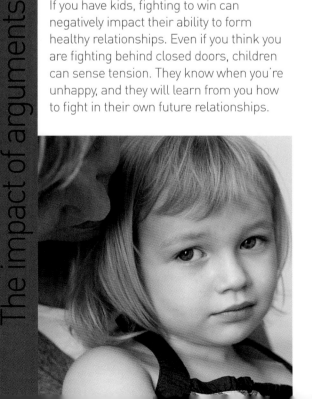

The impact of arguments

If you have kids, fighting to win can negatively impact their ability to form healthy relationships. Even if you think you are fighting behind closed doors, children can sense tension. They know when you're unhappy, and they will learn from you how to fight in their own future relationships.

How fighting affects kids

- **Fighting lowers self-esteem.** Kids who are surrounded by constant arguing often suffer from a lowered self-image and sense of self.
- **Fighting teaches fighting.** Being disagreeable is a learned behavior. Kids who witness selfish arguments (not healthy arguments) at home are much more likely to initiate disagreement or use anger to resolve problems in their own lives.
- **Fighting impacts success.** Children who deal with conflict at home are more likely to have difficulties in school and in other social situations.

In contrast, when you fight to love and come to a healthy resolution, you show your children how to communicate their anger and hurt in a way that is safe, fair, honest, and respectful.

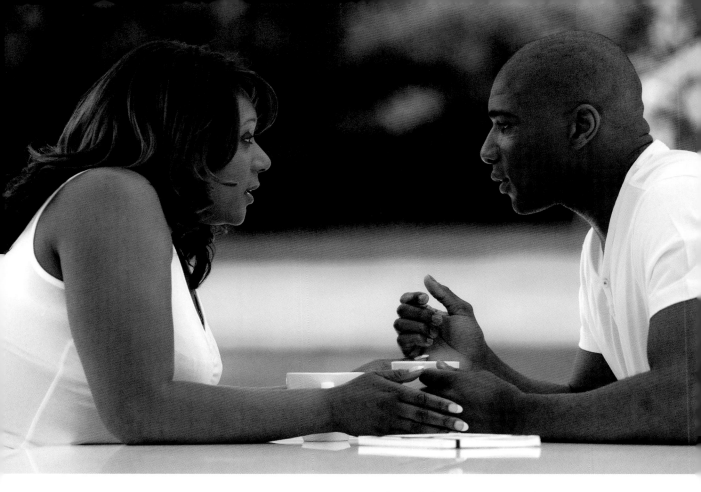

To take responsibility for your part of a conflict, it is important to own your 100 percent. This means accepting that you are the only one who can be held accountable for your life. In every relationship, each partner is 100 percent responsible for how they react to a given situation. When you own your part of a conflict, you empower yourself to shift things to where you'd like them to be.

It is especially important to take responsibility for your relationship when you feel like things have gotten off track. When this happens, sit down and really talk about what's going on. Agree that you can both call a "reboot" when the relationship hits a rough patch. This means deciding to stop harping on what has been going wrong, let go of blame and anger, and start with a clean slate, remembering that you are allies, not enemies, in your relationship.

Speaking unarguably

One of the best ways to fight well is to speak unarguably. When you do this, no one can disagree with you because you are only stating what is true for you. You are not making false accusations, and it is impossible for the opposite to be true (see page 19 for more on the question "Could the opposite be true?"). Speaking unarguably involves five main steps:

● Share a physical feeling, such as "I am feeling sick to my stomach," or "My chest hurts."
● Share an emotion from one of the five true emotions (anger, sadness, happiness, fear, and sexual attraction), such as "I feel sad and scared."
● Share the thoughts that inspire those feelings. "I feel sad because I think that you'd rather be with your friends than with me tonight."
● State a fact you know is true. For example, you

> **66** A win-win solution exists in every situation—you just have to stay open-minded enough to see it. **99**

can say, "I called you three times, but you didn't answer" instead of, "I called you three times, but you were too busy with your friends to answer."
- State what you want. For example, you might say: "I would like it if you would check in with me before you get in your car, so you won't have to answer your phone while you drive."
The fact is that you can only know what you are thinking and feeling, and this is what is useful to share with your partner. You can't speak unarguably using the word "you," because you don't know what your partner is thinking, so "I" statements are best. For example, instead of saying, "You never help me clean the house," you can say, "I feel angry when I have to clean the house alone." Or instead of saying, "You don't make me feel special," you can say, "I want to feel attractive and important to you." Speaking in this way lets you own your 100 percent and turn a fight into a productive conversation.

Communicating clearly

Arguments often deteriorate because one or both partners interpret something incorrectly. One way to avoid this is to practice repeating the statements that your partner makes to be sure that you understand. You can also mirror his statements, reflecting back what he is saying in a way that makes his desires clear to both of you. For example:

He says: When you turn me down in the bedroom, I feel embarrassed and unattractive.
You repeat: You are telling me that when I turn you down in the bedroom you feel embarrassed and unattractive.

You mirror: You take my refusal as a sign that I don't love you or find you desirable.

Statements like these will minimize arguments, and will help you reach a healthy resolution. They also prevent defensiveness, and protect you from saying hurtful things that will be hard to forgive.

Finding the win-win

Another key element in a healthy fight is focusing on finding the win-win solution. This exists in every situation—you just have to stay open-minded and let go of your need to be right in order to find it. For instance, perhaps you are arguing because his favorite team is playing on your date night, and he has been hinting that he'd like to watch it with his friends. If you're fighting to win in this situation, you might get angry and accuse him of loving football or his friends more than you. You might also give him an unequivocal "no," feel like a victim, and ultimately land in a frustrating argument.

Or, you might choose to find the win-win. To do this, it helps to speak out loud, something like: "I hear that this is an important game that you don't want to miss. And I really want to take advantage of our babysitter and get some alone time with you. I wonder how we can both get what we want?"

Brainstorm together. Maybe you go out to dinner and then he meets his friends. Maybe you put the babysitter off until the next afternoon, and go on a romantic picnic that you wouldn't be able to do at night. In every conflict, there are so many possibilities for the win-win. You just have to let go of wanting to be the only winner in order to see them.

The art of compromise

Once you have committed to changing your fighting style, you will be more open to one of the most important parts of fighting to love: compromise. When you compromise, you agree to consider your partner's needs along with your own. This means that you believe that your partner's needs are as valuable and valid as your own, and that you can meet them without losing your power or abandoning your own needs.

Personalized compromise

Take a good look at what problems you and your partner tend to run into again and again. Are you always fighting about how often it's okay to spend time apart with friends? Or does tension seem to arise over who's doing more of the household chores? Figure out the main issues that cause disagreement, and, when you are outside the heat of an argument, consider compromises you can reach together.

Although these solutions won't be failsafe and will take some adjustment for both of you, thinking logically about where you experience conflict can help you put old arguments to rest and begin your relationship with a clean slate. Not all problems will be 100 percent fixable, but your attitude is always 100 percent under your control. Fix what problems you can, and accept what problems cannot be fixed. This is not only the key to a happy relationship, it is the key to a happy life.

The issue: He gets upset that you are never in the mood for sex, yet you always feel too tired.
The solution: First, take a good look at your habits and emotions. Is he right that you've shut out sex? If so, are you not interested because you are too tired at the end of the day? Or, are you struggling with low libido? (If the latter, see pages 242–245 on treating low desire.) Next, try to understand where your partner is coming from and then seek out a compromise. (Reading the box, right, will help you see why having an active sex life is so important.) Maybe you aren't in the mood at night after a long, exhausting day, but you feel more energetic in the morning when both of you are well-rested and cuddling in bed. Or, if you are not an early bird, leave the dishes for later and try initiating sex after dinner. The important thing is to find a time that works for you, when you are most likely to be in the mood. This will help you commit to initiating sex

and showing your partner that you want him. At the same time, his flexibility about when and where sex takes place is a good reminder for you about how much he loves and desires you.

The issue: You think he spends too much money on "silly" things like video games or fishing rods.
The solution: Money is one of the main things that couples fight about. In fact, this timeless problem can drive even the happiest couple apart, and that's why this is one issue you need to figure out as soon as possible. Set up a household budget and allow each of you some spending money to use as you please. You might consider his video games unnecessary or even irresponsible, but he probably thinks the same about your designer lipstick or handbag addiction. Money will always be a source of contention, even for the most financially secure couples, but it becomes less of an issue once you find a way to manage it that works for both of you.

The issue: He doesn't pay attention to you when he comes home from work.
The solution: First, take a step back and remember that your partner loves you and would never want to hurt your feelings or ignore you. Then, tackle the problem at hand. Clearly, he is retreating into himself in these moments. So what's the deal? Tune into what your partner isn't saying. It might be that his body language is informing you that he needs time alone to decompress after work. Rather than pouncing on him the minute he comes in the door, or overloading him with complaints about your day, give him time to unwind for an hour. While you find stress relief from venting about a bad day, he might find it by sitting alone quietly or watching the game. So, call a girlfriend to talk about your boss. By the time you are off the phone, he will be ready to return to planet earth and talk about the day.

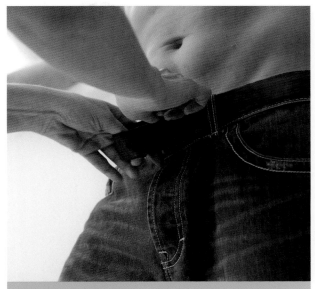

The truth about...

WHY MEN NEED SEX

If you're in a monogamous relationship and expect your partner to keep his commitment, it's important to remember that you are his only sexual outlet. This means it's patently unfair to shut down from sex. Owning and taking responsibility for this will go a long way toward having a healthy argument about sex and reaching a compromise that works for both of you.

In addition, although men typically are thought of as the initiators when it comes to sex, the truth is that they want to be pursued as well. They want to feel attractive and know that their partner enjoys them sexually—which means that if you are always turning him down or rarely initiate sex on your own, it will be hard for your partner not to take it personally. Think of it this way: Committing to sex is a way of committing to your partner and your relationship.

Putting your partner first

Part of the problem in putting your partner first is the idea of unconditional love. In a long-term relationship, you trust that your partner will always be there for you, which is something few people can say for their employer. Because of this, the temptation is always there to prioritize your career over your relationship, but it's important to remember that while love may be unconditional, relationship growth is not. You can only move forward to a more intimate, passionate, fun relationship when you put in the time and truly make your partner your number one priority.

Shutting off the office

Would you choose your smartphone over your spouse? According to a survey released by Sheraton Hotels & Resorts 87 percent of professionals admit to taking their phone into the bedroom with them, and an astounding 84 percent of respondents admit the first and last thing they do everyday is check their email. To top it all off, 35 percent of professionals admitted that, if forced to choose, they would pick their phone over their spouse! Those are pretty high numbers.

It might sound a little extreme, but just ask any iPhone widow or Blackberry divorcée. It is possible to be replaced by a phone. Think about it. How many dinners have you worked your way through? How many vacations have you phoned in? How many special moments with your spouse and family have you ignored as you frantically dial clients from home?

The lure of constantly being attached to the office is hard to resist. In today's uncertain economy, staying connected to the workplace and the needs of your employer seems like a must. However, while most professionals believe that being constantly available is a requirement for career advancement, it can actually be more hurtful than beneficial if you don't erect at least some boundaries. When you are constantly plugged-in—checking your email status, working on projects, and speaking with clients well into the night—you never get a chance to rest. This not only affects you physically, but also emotionally, intellectually, and in your relationship. Your creativity and emotional insight suffer from lack of mental rest, and so does your connection with your partner. So what is the solution?

Commit to balance. Successful athletes follow a "rest-and-recover" model. Muscles actually develop during times of rest, not training. Thus, without days off, muscles never have a chance to reach their full potential. Additionally, they become strained and can tear due to overuse. The same is true for mental exercise—so unplug. Put the phone on silent. Leave your reports at the office. Take a walk, cook dinner, talk to your kids, read a good book. Do what you enjoy, at least for an hour a day. A balanced life is a healthy life.

Enjoy romance for romance's sake. Too often people use romance as a means to an end. Spend a little time this week merely enjoying romance for the sake of it. Share a bottle of wine with your spouse. Enjoy a hot bath. Have a couple's massage. Don't do these things with an end goal in mind—simply focus on each other and enjoy the moment.

Pull the plug on technology. No, really. If you can't go cold turkey, try turning off your phone for at least a couple of hours each day. Then, try and go a whole Sunday without logging in once. Unplug every

> 66 There are lots of ways to unplug from work—you just need to find the one that works for you. 99

night at 6 PM or commit to putting your phone away on the weekends. Or, make an agreement with your partner that your phones will be turned off during any time that you spend alone together (which for most of us is rare). There are lots of options—you just need to find the one that for works for you and that allows you to enjoy downtime the most.

The benefits of "choreplay"

Don't rely on French maid costumes. If you want to increase the amount of sex in your relationship, hand the duster to your man! A recent survey in *Parenting* magazine found that 15 percent of women are aroused when their partners pitch in around the house, also known as "choreplay."

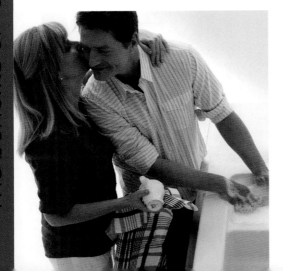

How housework can amount to more sex

Additionally, a 2006 study found that men who helped with household chores were more attractive to their spouses. Why is this? Aside from the fact that some of us simply enjoy the sight of a man in an apron, it could be that women are turned on by choreplay because it gives us a chance to take a much-needed break, and reminds us that we are in a marriage of equals. Even though most women now work outside the home, many of us still perform the bulk of household chores and responsibilities. So men, listen up: cleaning the house unasked is one of the best ways to put your partner first—and can also get you some extra action in the bedroom (a win-win solution if ever there was one.)

TOP 5

RELATIONSHIP MISCONCEPTIONS

Sometimes couples get into arguments because they have different expectations about what being in love should look like and feel like. When you compare your relationship with the relationships of people around you, or the ones you see portrayed in movies or on television, you can end up buying into a lot of misconceptions about what a successful, loving partnership should look like. Being aware of these misconceptions and having healthy expectations will go a long way toward preventing arguments and keeping your relationship peaceful.

1 Everyone else is having more sex than us.

People often assume that everyone around them is indulging in wild sexual activity. The truth is that, on average, long-term couples have sex once a week. If you are unhappy with your current sex life, you shouldn't ignore your feelings, but make sure that your unhappiness doesn't stem from unrealistic comparisons.

2 Now that I am part of a couple, I need to let go of the "single" me.

While it is important to make your partner number one in your life, time spent developing your own interests is still a good thing. Absence makes the heart grow fonder—and even more important, it gives you time to explore yourself and develop new ideas, keeping you happy, energized, and interesting.

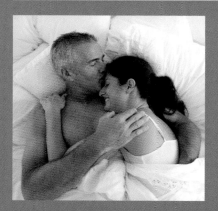

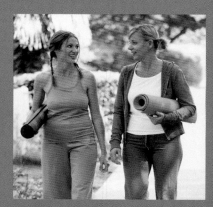

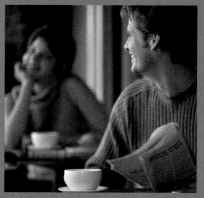

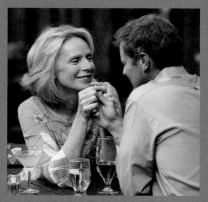

3 I am not allowed to find other people attractive.

The truth is that there is no reason why committed couples shouldn't notice attractive people. After all, you are still living, breathing, sexual beings! Once you acknowledge the attraction, it will likely lose its grip on you. Then, you can channel that increased awareness of the power of seduction into your own relationship.

4 Our kids should always come first.

This sounds good on paper, but in practice, it means that you and your partner never get the TLC you need to keep your relationship strong. Showing your kids what a loving relationship looks like is a precious gift, so make sure that you create time for date night and adult-only events and vacations on a regular basis.

5 I have to do it all or it won't get done.

Women especially often feel like this because we are prone to want things to look a certain way in order to feel content. However, if you do everything for your partner, you infantilize him and turn yourself into a harried, frenzied mess. Let him take care of you sometimes. After all, that's what a true partnership is all about!

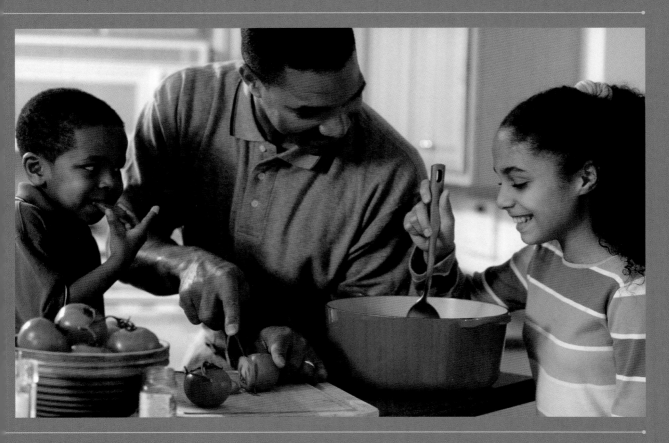

Intimacy and sex

Have you ever noticed that when your sex life goes awry, your relationship tends to go awry as well? For example, when sex dwindles, do you notice that your partner seems less invested in you, or less affectionate? This isn't all in your head! When your sex life takes a hit, it often has a ripple effect throughout your relationship, and it can impact your communication, your intimacy, and your happiness.

The sex and intimacy link

Sex and intimacy are closely linked in our brains; however, men and women respond differently to intimacy. Many men have trouble feeling emotionally intimate with their partner when they can't connect with her sexually. At the same time, most women can't get in the mood or enjoy sex without that intimate connection. For men, sex feeds intimacy, and for women, intimacy feeds sex.

Thus, when your sex life goes off the rails, you might find that your partner isn't as emotionally intimate as normal. He might not call you by your pet name or offer you as much affection or notice when you take the trouble to make him a special dinner. Ironically, by neglecting to do these things, he is not providing the connection and romance you need to feel sexual. Sound familiar? It's a vicious cycle and one that can get out of hand if you don't tend to it quickly.

Maintaining sex and intimacy

This might seem obvious, but one of the best ways to ensure that the sex and intimacy cycle doesn't unravel is to have regular sex. Even if you aren't in the mood, try to have a "just do it" philosophy (assuming there's no serious physical or emotional issue stopping you, of course). The more you have sex, the more you will want to have sex—and the better you will get at it! Orgasms will come more easily and inhibitions will decrease. Even more importantly, you will find that the more frequently you have sex with your partner, the closer and more intimate your relationship will be.

At the same time, when you aren't getting the affection or intimacy you need, don't be afraid to spell it out for your partner. Choose not to get upset or feel neglected about his lack of attention. Instead, realize that trusting your partner (a requirement for any successful relationship) means trusting his love

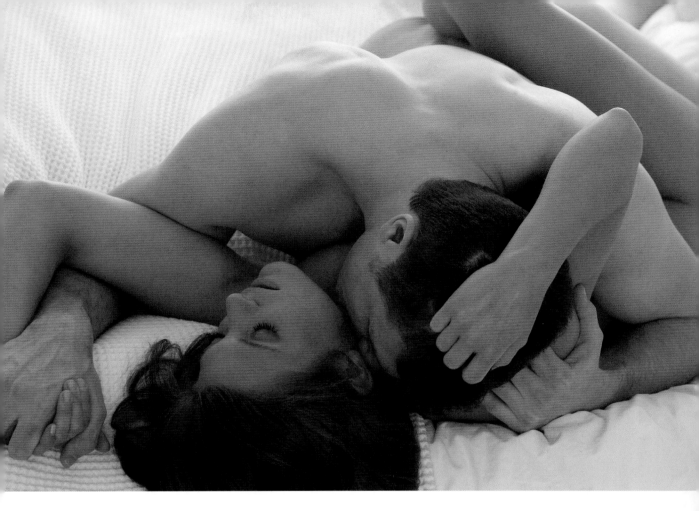

for you even when you aren't feeling it. The best way to turn the relationship in the direction you want it to go is to speak his language and tell him directly what you need. For example, you might say: "I love it when you kiss me passionately" or, "I feel so special when you plan a romantic date for us."

You both have distinct needs that must be met in order to develop a healthy relationship. Sometimes this means that you have to be vocal about your needs so your partner can meet them, while other times it means accepting your partner's different genetic makeup and prioritizing sex. Men might not be from Mars, but they certainly approach relationships differently from women, and this is something you have to understand and accept in order to build a truly intimate relationship.

The truth about...

THE IMPACT OF LESS SEX

When sex isn't working, our non-sexual physical intimacy breaks down and our threshold for getting angry with each other becomes much lower. This means that there is very little handholding, kissing, cuddling, or other types of intimate touch—sometimes dangerously none at all. It also means that little things that shouldn't matter can lead to huge arguments. All of this highlights the importance of committing to a healthy sex life along with healthy communication.

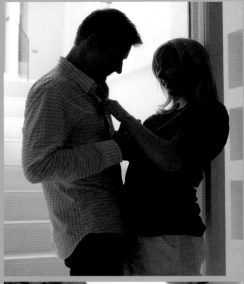

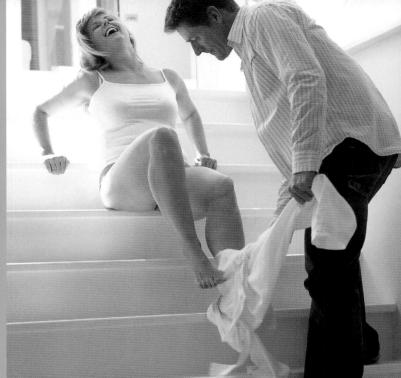

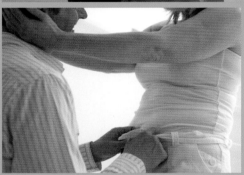

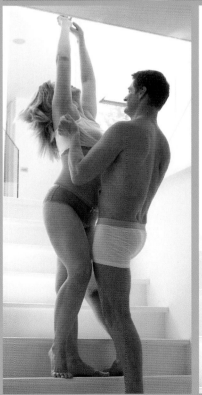

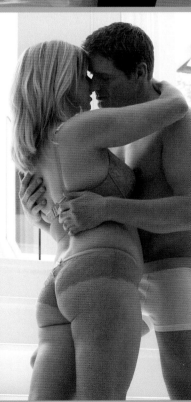

Strip down

Add a bit of fun and spontaneity to intimacy by undressing each other pre-sex. Start slowly, removing one piece of clothing at a time, and reveling in each new bit of skin revealed and ready to be touched. Increase seduction levels by starting this game in a new part of the house—try the stairs, the living room, the kitchen—building anticipation and sexual thrill as you move toward the intimate climax of the bedroom.

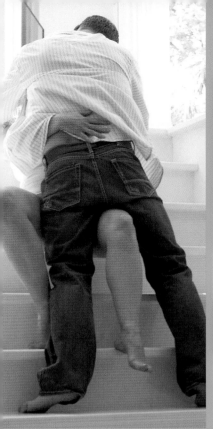
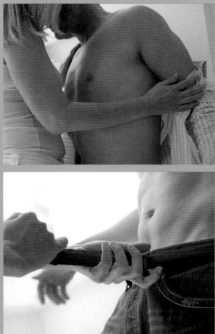
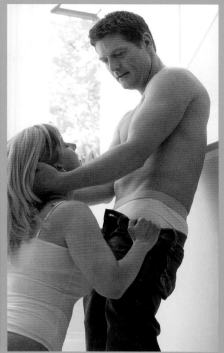
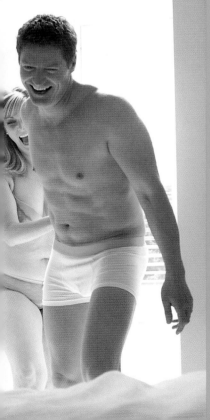
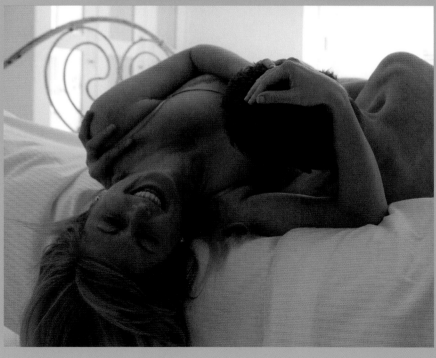

Avoiding the major trouble spots

Dr. John Gottman, the famous marriage and relationship researcher and therapist, once outlined the four signs that a marriage is headed for failure based on his research observing hundreds of couples. He called these signs the "Four Horsemen of the Apocalypse," and they are behaviors that we exhibit during arguments or times of stress. However, we can also exhibit these behaviors long after the argument is over, carrying around silent stress and tension.

Trouble #1: Criticism

There is nothing wrong with expressing your needs or feelings to your partner, even if—sometimes especially if—they are not harmonious feelings. However, the way that you deliver these feelings is very important. If you are being critical, then you are in Apocalypse territory. When you criticize your partner, you attack his personality and his self-worth. In contrast, when you offer feedback, you simply voice your feelings about a behavior or an incident. Offering feedback means that you aren't insulting, attacking, or going on the offensive. You'll see the difference in the examples below.

Criticism: "You are so lazy! I guess I will have to cut the grass by myself, as usual."
Feedback: "Can you please cut the grass? I feel angry when you don't, because it makes me feel like I'm on my own and have no one to help me."

Criticism: "Do you ever think before you talk? My sister is going to be pouting for the next month about your inconsiderate comment!"
Feedback: "I know you were only joking, but my sister doesn't have very thick skin. Can you please apologize to her so we can all be on good terms again?"

Criticism: "Late from work again, huh? I guess we know what's most important to you."
Feedback: "I am sorry you have been working so late, but can you please call me next time you are going to be late, so I don't worry about you?"

Before you slip into criticism, remember that you don't know what your partner is thinking or feeling, so you shouldn't be using statements that rely on "you." Instead, speak unarguably (for more on this, see page 178), and use "I" statements, to make sure that you are offering feedback instead of criticism.

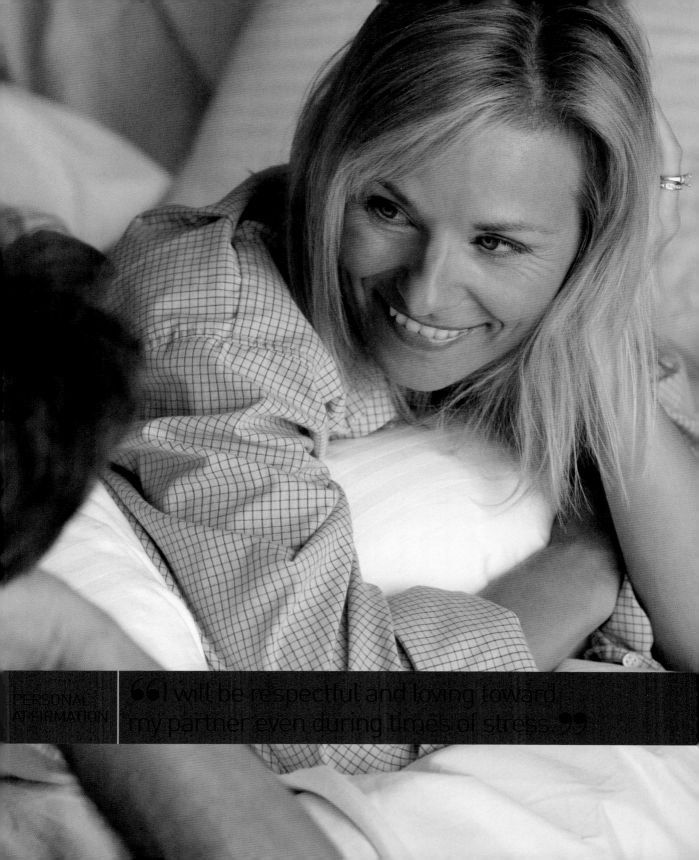

PERSONAL
AFFIRMATION

"I will be respectful and loving toward my partner even during times of stress "

> **66** When you are open to your partner's vulnerabilities, you will be able to build an honest partnership. **99**

Trouble #2: Contempt

Much like criticism, contempt cuts at the heart of a person's feelings and sense of self. Contempt is wounding, useless, and very hard to move past and forgive. When you are behaving contemptuously, you might roll your eyes, mock your partner, name-call, or act in other ways that are insulting. All of these symptoms show that you are judging your partner and disregarding his feelings, which means that you are no longer allies. Some examples of contemptuous statements include:

- "Why don't you get up off the couch and exercise?"
- "Nice outfit! Are you trying to embarrass me?"
- "I can't believe you chose this restaurant. What a joke. The food is awful!"
- "I hate your friends. How can you stand such jerks?"

When we read these expressions of contempt in black and white, it is hard to believe that anyone would say such cruel things to their partner. And yet we do, sometimes in the heat of the moment, sometimes because we are "joking," and sometimes because we are sad and upset, but don't know how to express it except through anger. Contempt is deadly in a relationship, and it must be completely eradicated.

Make it a point to do this by telling your partner that you want to "reboot" the relationship. If you have reacted with contempt in the past, acknowledge this, and say that you want to recommit to being on the same page. Then, ask your partner to help you change. Have him repeat things that he finds contemptuous, and listen to his feedback. Remember, if it hurts his feelings, it needs to be removed from your communication, even if it seems harmless to you.

Trouble #3: Defensive behavior

The third horseman of the apocalypse is defensive behavior. When you are defensive, you are trapped by your need to be right. Much like it sounds, defensive behavior is straight out of a sports game. You want to win, you want to challenge your partner, and you want to get bragging rights. Not exactly the behavior of someone who is fighting to love! Some examples of defensive behavior include:

- "I told you to pick up the cleaning after work. I am 100 percent sure that I did, because I remember thinking that you would probably forget."
- "I am not the one who said we would go to this party. You were, remember? I certainly do!"
- "It's not my fault the puppy peed on the carpet. I told you the kids weren't going to take responsibility for it! Why are you blaming me?"

Even if the above statements were all true, the person saying those things would still be far from "right" in the true sense of what that word means in a relationship. It doesn't ultimately matter if you give your partner good advice that he ignores, or if he forgets something that you asked him to do. The real question is: Would you rather be "right" or be in love? No one wants to be with someone who won't accept fault for anything.

You will recognize how toxic defensiveness can be once you connect with the fact that you are 100 percent responsible for your life. Defensive behavior is a useless and even dishonest way to behave. When you let go of this habit, you will be more open to your partner's vulnerabilities, and will be able to build a more honest and productive partnership.

Trouble #4: Stonewalling

The last horseman of the Apocalypse, stonewalling is perhaps the most painful and also the most pervasive. This is the favorite behavior of those of us who tend to be passive aggressive. If you have passive aggressive tendencies, you are uncomfortable expressing anger, you prefer to avoid conflict, and you are rarely direct about what you want and need. This is especially common with women, as many of us grew up never learning to embrace and express anger, or ask for what we want.

A good way to identify stonewalling is this: If you mentally or physically remove yourself from your partner and his needs, you are stonewalling, which also means you are shutting him out. When you stonewall, it might seem like you are choosing not to argue, but you are actually choosing not to engage. Some examples of stonewalling include:

● You are upset about a comment your partner made. However, when your partner asks you what's wrong, you sharply say, "Nothing," and leave it at that.

● Your partner is angry that you overdrew the checking account again. When he asks you about where the money went, you leave and go for a walk.

● Your partner asks why you refuse to go to his family's holiday celebration. Instead of telling him that it's because his brother hurt your feelings last year, you shrug it off and say you don't want to go.

The truth is that avoidance won't make the problem go away. In fact, it generally makes the situation more rife with hurt and anger. By refusing to communicate, you are doing as much damage as if you were screaming or throwing things. Instead, open up to your partner by speaking unarguably. You don't have to express your deepest fears, but you can say, "I feel sad when I call you at work and you speak so brusquely to me." Address your immediate feelings and stay in the present. Sharing this little bit of emotion can help improve your communication and stop stonewalling in its tracks.

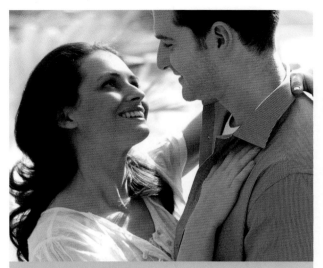

How to...

VOICE APPRECIATION

One of the best ways to protect your relationship is to be purposeful about telling your partner the things you love about him. Keeping appreciation constant in your relationship protects against all the major trouble spots we've discussed. Here's how.

1 Large or small, express appreciation to your partner every day. When you live in a spirit of gratitude, you and your relationship will be happier and healthier.

2 Be specific. Instead of saying, "I appreciate you for being a good father," say "I appreciate when you spend time playing with the kids at night. It gives me a few moments to regroup" or "I appreciate that you picked up the dog food we needed. I was dreading going to the store and now I don't have to. Thank you."

3 Tell your partner three things you appreciate about him every day—I challenge you! He will be blown away by your love and approval, and will ultimately learn to express appreciation to you, too.

Dealing with economic disparity

In today's era of gender equality, sometimes nothing is more nerve-wracking than the arrival of the check at the end of a dinner date. Who should pay? Where does romance end and equality begin? These same struggles can apply to long-term couples on a grander scale. One thing's for sure: Whether you are single or part of a couple, knowing how to manage money is a key part of the modern relationship.

Salary and gender

Traditionally, as we all know, men have been the breadwinners. However, in our current economic setting some women may be earning more than the men in their lives. According to a recent analysis of 2005 US census data, young women in urban environments such as New York, Chicago, and Boston are earning higher wages than men in the same age range. This income gap may be due to the fact that women in their 20s are more likely than their male counterparts to have college degrees and graduate degrees, which translate to larger salaries.

While all of this may be one large leap for womankind, many women are finding that earning more money is an obstacle to love. Unfortunately, even the most enlightened man can sometimes feel intimidated by a woman who has a higher salary. So, how can you navigate this new gender challenge?

Forgo the awkwardness that occurs when the check arrives by agreeing that whoever asks should pay. This will allow each of you to feel comfortable at the restaurant of your choice.

Never discuss money on a first date—or a second or a third. Wait until you know you are both interested and want to consider a more serious relationship. Money should not become an issue until you are in a committed, long-term partnership. At that point, understanding both of your financial limits will help you develop a system that works for both of you.

Abandon traditional gender roles. Some men feel so intimidated by a high-earning partner that they are unable to perform in the bedroom. To these men I say—get over it! Let go of traditional roles and embrace gender freedom, both inside and outside the bedroom. Most importantly, appreciate your partner's intelligence and ambition.

And by the way, did you hear that sound? It is the sound of the glass ceiling cracking from the boardroom to the bedroom! Congratulations to the hard-working, large-earning women who are beginning to reign in our cities.

Protecting your partner's pride

While women should never be ashamed of their earning potential, if you earn more than your partner it's important to be purposeful about letting him be a man. This is especially true if he decides to stay at home with the kids while you focus on your career. Even if you are both happy with this arrangement, your partner may still sometimes struggle with insecurities that he is not acting as your family's primary financial provider.

Encouraging your partner to make decisions about your life and how you spend your money together will help him feel good about himself, and will keep him involved in the relationship. Nurturing his masculine energy in this way also protects your attraction to him. Read on for ways to provide support, and to ensure that both of you feel like you're contributing equally to your relationship.

Don't turn him into Mr. Mom. Even if your partner is taking care of the kids, that doesn't mean you should expect him to take over all the household duties. Regardless of who is the stay-at-home partner, it's important that you each help around the house to make sure that no one ends up feeling like he or she is doing a thankless job.

Appreciate him. Appreciation is always important, but it can be more important than ever when you abandon traditional roles. Make sure to vocalize how smart, caring, and patient you find your partner. Cite specific things that he does well, whether it's helping the kids with homework or cutting the lawn.

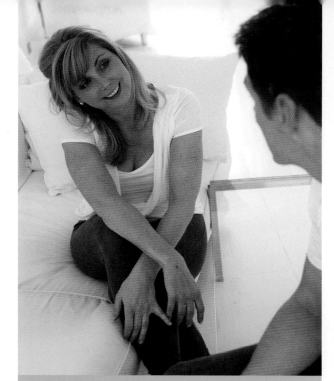

The truth about...

DEALING WITH UNEMPLOYMENT

Most of us are worriers by nature, but it is best not to panic or despair if your partner loses his job. Letting fear get out of control does not help either of you. Of course, this is not to say that you should hide your concerns or pretend everything is fine. Talking honestly about how you're feeling is important, but so is carefully and calmly going over your options.

As you do this, listen. It's easy to offer trite advice like "You will find something," but remember, your partner probably hears advice like this all day long. The truth is that there is nothing you can really say that will make him feel better, but you can support him by listening, mirroring his statements (for more on this, see page 179), and offering encouragement and love. For example, when he says, "I am so angry right now. I know I will never find a job!" you can say, "You are angry and scared right now. You feel like everything is out of control. How can I support you?"

Overcoming infidelity

Is infidelity a forgivable sin? When surveyed, 90 percent of Americans say that infidelity is wrong, yet 20 percent of men and 13 percent of women actually do cheat on their spouses. Infidelity is devastating families across the country, and the cycle of self-blame, betrayal, and anger can be difficult to break. The good news, however, is that if you seek help early and confront the issues that instigated the affair, you can recover your relationship.

Dealing with blame

After an affair, it is common for both partners to feel that the other is to blame. In order for healing to begin, each partner must explore the personal issues that may have contributed to the infidelity. Sometimes, cheating may be a symptom of a larger midlife crisis where the adulterer is questioning everything in his or her life, including work, marriage, and friendships. Other times, there is a family history of infidelity, and cheating was actually a "learned behavior" reinforced at home.

It is also possible that the betrayed partner had withdrawn from the relationship, been overly critical, or become emotionally unavailable. Ultimately, like sex, infidelity is always a couple's issue. Once there is some clarity about what issues each partner has brought to the table, you can start to work on repairing the relationship.

Beginning recovery

There is no quick fix for recovering after an affair, but I encourage couples that are recovering from this extreme trauma to commit to therapy every week for a while. I also suggest that the couple make an adultery contract, stating the adulterer's promise not to cheat again and to cut off all contact with the affair. In addition, the adulterer should regularly assure the betrayed partner that there has been no contact with the person involved in the affair. If this person tries to contact him or her, the adulterer must report that the contact was not accepted or returned.

It is also important to avoid having long periods of time for which you aren't accountable. A couple recovering from an affair should know each other's schedules more closely than they did before the affair occurred. This will help ease the mind of the betrayed partner, who is often plagued with thoughts of the affair. Feelings of depression, worthlessness, and extreme anger are common.

The victim should be able to vent his or her anger, but in a controlled, time-limited way. It is difficult for the relationship to heal if you are constantly reliving the past. I advise couples to allow 10 minutes a day for venting. The victim can take this time whenever he or she wants, and can scream and throw emotional darts, but only for a short, defined period.

The betrayed spouse should also be able to ask questions, and the adulterer should answer them. However, you should avoid giving the gory sexual details, which will not help with healing down the road. If questions become too sexually specific, you can gently remind your partner that the details won't contribute to getting your relationship back on track. If pressured, you can answer honestly but generally. For example, you might say, "Yes, we had sex four times in the course of the affair," instead of, "We had sex in every possible position."

Renewing physical intimacy

Sex is often more challenging after an affair. Both partners think about the affair during sex, and emotional vulnerabilities run high. The betrayed partner might be thinking about how he or she measures up to the affair, while the adulterous partner may also have some sexual difficulties arising from feelings of guilt and shame, or even from fantasizing about the affair.

The truth is that sexual healing can only begin after a measure of forgiveness has been achieved. A couple must rebuild their sexual relationship from the ground up. Much of the work involves communicating to build a relationship where there is equal power in and outside of the bedroom. Forgiving infidelity is a difficult process, but it never ceases to amaze me how marriages can actually thrive after an affair. Infidelity is a life-changing event for both partners, but once they do the work, on themselves and their relationship, their marriage can become stronger and closer than before.

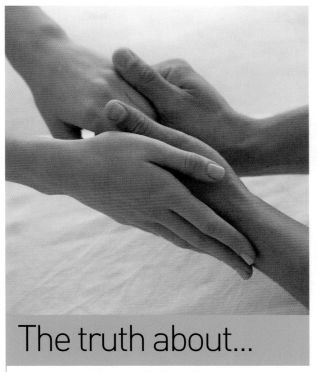

The truth about...

CLOSE CO-ED RELATIONSHIPS

Humans are sexual beings, and I truly believe that it is almost impossible for a heterosexual man and woman to be completely devoid of sexual thoughts or wishes on one side or the other. Friendship already indicates a level of attraction and affection, which can lead to gray areas. This isn't to say that men and women can't ever be friends, but it's important to be realistic about how flirtation can be a risk. Ultimately, you have to decide what constitutes infidelity in your relationship. For example, maybe you can both have friends of the opposite sex, but can't hang out one-on-one with that person. The rules can be as strict or as liberal as you choose, as long as you and your partner are both comfortable with them.

The happiness experiment

If you really want to put the kibosh on any resentment in your relationship, I encourage you to consider what may feel like a radical experiment: agree with your partner to wholeheartedly and consciously put each other's happiness first. This means putting your own needs and desires aside and really thinking about what makes your partner happy. Ideally, you should commit to this experiment for a week, but you can also try it for just a few days.

The terms of happiness

The idea of this experiment is that you each make a verbal and emotional commitment to put the other's happiness first—above what you want, what you need, and even what you think will make you happy in that moment. Of course, a plan like this requires commitment and trust that each of you will follow through. When this happens, the results can be truly life- and relationship-changing. I've tried this in my own relationship and have had numerous couples try it out as well. Invariably, there are positive results. What always seems to happen is that the act of giving and loving and putting your partner first requires that you put your ego away—and that feels really good. When you do this, you also land much more naturally at the win-win solution without getting defensive.

I know it feels scary to consider putting your own needs on the back burner for your partner. If you are hesitant, remember two things. First, the experiment is for a short period of time, not forever. Second, your partner is committing to the same thing. Even more important, what you'll find as you start on this journey is that if you really follow through, you'll both be happy and little details like these won't matter any more.

Practicing selflessness

Here's how it works: In any given situation throughout the experiment, you should express your needs and desires. Don't feel like you need to become a puppet, agreeing with everything your partner says. However—and here's the important part—after you have expressed your needs, really listen to your partner and respect his needs and desires. You absolutely should still state what you want, but then you should do what will make him happy. In return, he should be making every effort to do what makes you happy.

For example, if your partner says he'd like to go to an action film rather than the romantic comedy you were thinking of, you might say, "I was thinking I'd like to see that romantic comedy, but your happiness is most important, so let's go to the action film." Nine times out of ten, his defenses will be completely down and he will find it so easy to respond that he will decide to vote for the romantic comedy because your happiness is most important to him. In fact, that's the best part of this experiment—rather than feeling as though you're always succumbing to your partner's needs, you both will invariably (and easily) get your way much more often than usual.

Or, maybe he wants to let the kids stay a second night at their friend's house, but you're worried they'll be too tired. You can say, "I'm worried the kids will be exhausted spending another night, but if it makes you happy, I'm okay with it." Your partner will then likely stop for a minute and consider, "Does this really make me happy? Maybe she's right. Anyway, her happiness is most important to me, so let's have the kids come home."

The long-term effect

As you practice this experiment, you will be surprised at how romantic and spontaneous your relationship becomes. In fact, you may be reminded of those early days of dating, when you were eager to please each other. Instead of obsessing about getting what you want, you will be able to let go and trust that your partner will meet your needs. Once you focus on the give and not the take, you will be surprised by how natural it becomes, how satisfying it is, and how much happier you and your partner are together.

Happiness protection

There is one caveat to the happiness experiment: If what makes your partner happy is against your morals or feels scary, then you shouldn't put his happiness first. Obviously, if what would make him happy is to rob a bank together or have sex eight times a day, then he's not doing his part by putting your happiness first.

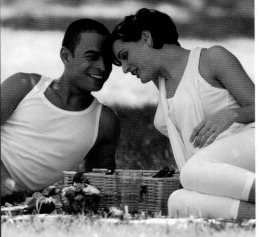

Finding a compromise

If your partner asks you to engage in something that makes you uncomfortable (for example, a threesome), you can simply say, "I am not able to do that, but I hear that you want to do something spontaneous and different. I want to make you happy, so let's find some way that we can accomplish that." (For the record, I never think threesomes are a good idea unless you have an open or polyamorous relationship, superhuman levels of emotional maturity, and not a jealous bone in your body.)

Bottom line? The whole point of this experiment is that you are both putting the other person first; therefore, once you express your dismay, fear, or discomfort, your partner should automatically back off and find a new idea. If he doesn't, then he isn't playing by the rules.

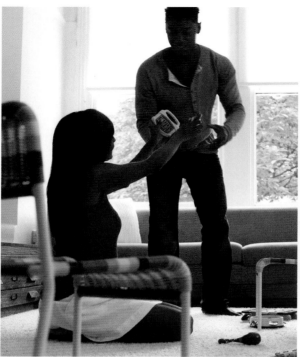
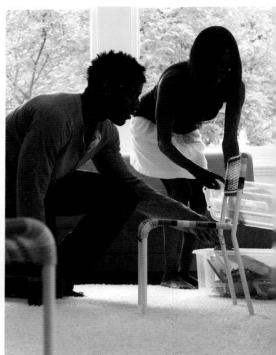

Chapter 8

Juggling family and relationships

Few things bring more joy than family, but it is also true that few things bring more stress. Finding the right level of involvement with in-laws can be a huge challenge, particularly when kids enter the picture. Navigate family relationships successfully by creating space for regular alone-time with your partner and finding time for the hobbies and friendships that make you uniquely *you*.

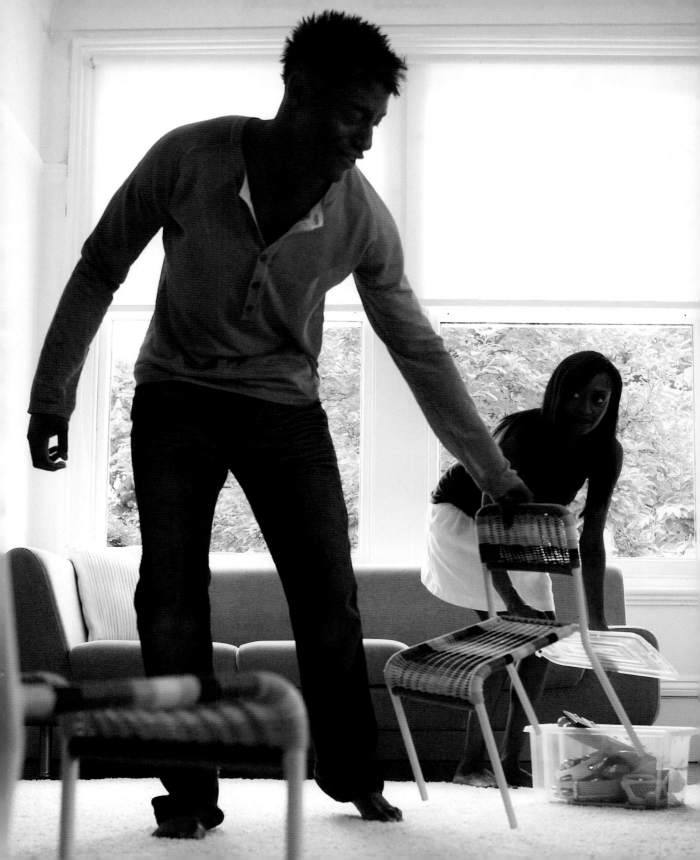

Every woman in every relationship finds it difficult to manage her romantic life with her life as a daughter, sister, friend, and employee. Time is valuable, and it never feels like we have enough. This is especially true when it comes to balancing time with your partner and your family, who can often be demanding in their requests, whether or not they mean to be. Take this quiz to evaluate how you manage your time. Then, read on to find ways to increase the time you devote to the most important thing—your relationship.

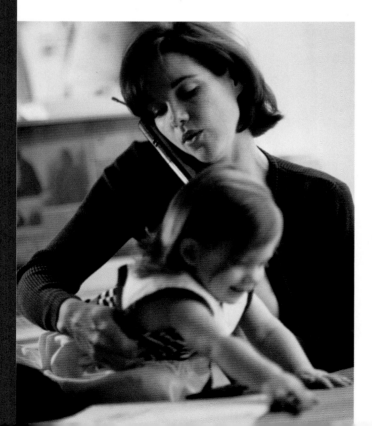

1 YOUR PARTNER MADE RESERVATIONS AT ONE of the most exclusive restaurants in town. You are really looking forward to going, but you can't help feeling guilty about leaving the kids with a new babysitter. To compromise, you:
Ⓐ Bring your kids with you. The other diners won't mind!
Ⓑ Ask the babysitter to call you if anything goes wrong, and leave the number of the restaurant for her.
Ⓒ Cancel your dinner. The kids come first, and you can always plan a date for another night.

2 YOUR FRIEND WANTS YOU TO JOIN A GYM WITH HER. Even though your life is hectic right now, you really want to get in shape and fit back into your skinny jeans, so you tell her that you'll:
Ⓐ Buy an expensive package complete with training sessions. You might not follow through with your plan, but it's worth it to have access to the coolest gym in town.
Ⓑ Schedule time to work out during your lunch hour, so you can exercise while still managing all of your other responsibilities at home and work.
Ⓒ Skip it. You have way too much going on to squeeze in the gym.

3 YOU ARE TRYING TO LAND A BIG PROMOTION AT WORK. It is stressful and you don't have much time to spend at home with the kids. The morning of your big presentation, your daughter comes down with the chicken pox. You:

A Promise to bring her chicken noodle soup on your way home from work, kiss her goodbye, and race out the door so you won't be late.

B Ask your partner to take care of her during the morning so you can give your presentation, and then swap during the afternoon. After all your hard work, an afternoon of Disney movies and quality time with your daughter will be rejuvenating, chicken pox notwithstanding!

C Postpone your presentation and rush around the house disinfecting everything so your youngest child doesn't get the chicken pox, too.

4 IT'S CHRISTMAS TIME, AND YOU ARE HOSTING

your in-laws for a few days. Between present wrapping, cookie baking, and keeping the kids from killing each other, your nerves are frayed. To release the stress, you:

A End up getting into a screaming match with your partner, calling him lazy and telling him to finish the Christmas shopping since you have done everything else.

B Ask your in-laws to help babysit the kids so you can finish wrapping your presents, and send your partner to the store to buy last-minute tree trimmings in your stead.

C Relax? You won't be able to take a break until after New Year's Eve!

5 IT'S LATE AT NIGHT, AND YOU AND YOUR PARTNER

are starting to get intimate for the first time in weeks. However, you hear the pitter patter of little feet, and realize that one of your kids is awake and coming down the hall. You:

A Panic and throw on clothes, then snap at your partner when he wants to just shout to your son that you'll be right there. Even though it's usually nothing, what if he really needs you?

B Thank God you put a lock on the bedroom door. Take your kid back to bed, and then come back to finish what you started.

C Let your child sleep between you and your partner. It's the only way any of you will get any rest.

6 YOU HAVE RECENTLY SWITCHED CAREER PATHS,

and are now earning more than your partner. He is happy for you, but you suspect he may also feel slightly inadequate. To find out, you:

A Tease him about how you are now the breadwinner in the family. If he has any insecurites about this, surely he'll bring them up.

B Make time after dinner one night to enjoy a glass of wine and talk over any concerns either of you have about your recent lifestyle changes.

C Offer to give up your new job if he would prefer.

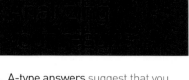

A-type answers suggest that you certainly know how to take time for yourself and meet your most immediate needs. However, you often do so at the expense of other's needs, and your hectic schedule makes you feel grumpy and entitled. This is not a healthy way to multi-task, and will likely impact the happiness of your relationship.

B-type answers indicate that you are probably pretty adept at juggling all your responsibilities in a way that works best for you, your relationship, and your family. You make your needs a priority, but also are open to making sacrifices to meet the needs of your loved ones.

C-type answers mean that you likely have trouble making time for yourself and your own needs. Although it might seem heroic to constantly cater to your family, this causes you to build up resentment and will eventually lead to a blowout. A healthier approach is to admit when you don't have time to do something, and make sure to find time for things that make you happy.

> 66 Every woman finds it hard to manage her romantic life with her life as a daughter, sister, and friend. 99

Transitioning from couple to family

Once you and your partner begin a family, you will notice that your roles inevitably shift. Not only will you look and feel different physically, you will also feel different emotionally, and you will want different things. Happy hour with your co-workers may seem unappealing in comparison to a nap, and shopping for a new pair of shoes seems unimportant when compared to the excitement of spending some quality time with your little one. These are all good changes; it just takes a period of adjustment to acclimate to your exciting new life.

Staying close

Transitioning into your new roles as parents often brings unexpected stressors, and it is common for couples to fight during this time. There are many reasons for this. Despite his excitement, your partner might feel jealous because the baby is taking so much of your time and attention. Or, you might feel resentful that your partner isn't helping more with the late night feedings. Remember that you are both exhausted and overwhelmed. Knowing that everyone encounters these fears and frustrations will help you to feel less frightened and alone.

Get practical and work out a schedule you can both agree to for the feedings, diaper changes, and other new responsibilities. This way you are both more likely to get the rest you need. Even more importantly, remember that you are allies in this new journey. People often talk about how amazing and life-changing parenting is, but that doesn't mean that it isn't also frustrating, difficult, and even temporarily unrewarding. Discussing these challenges and being honest about your feelings rather than behaving like nothing is wrong will help keep you bonded to your partner.

Your sexual connection

Along with parenting challenges such as stress or lack of time, you might find that you are struggling to feel sexy or desirable after childbirth. Many women struggle because they feel like a "mom," someone who is there to buy juice boxes, make beds, and drive kids around all day. They don't feel in touch with their inner vixens, and their libido suffers as a result. When you don't feel sexually attractive, you aren't going to be interested in sex. Realizing that you can be both the sexy vixen and the caring mother will help you transition into this complex new role more smoothly. (For more on how to do this, see pages 144–145.)

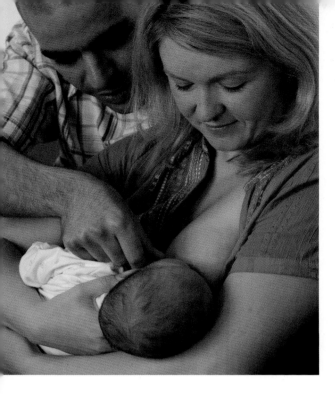

In addition, there are some physical effects of childbirth that can complicate sex. The vagina might be too tight after an episiotomy, and scar tissue from labor can make it inflexible, which means that intercourse may be painful for you at first. Internal adhesions from a C-section—especially multiple C-sections—can also make sex hurt. It's always important to get to the bottom of these physical concerns with a doctor who listens to you and offers you options for treating them.

Along with your own personal difficulties adjusting to a post-baby sex life, you may find your partner suddenly has a hard time viewing you as a sexual object. We often hear about the plummeting hormones, body-image issues, and sleep deprivation that plague new mothers, but rarely do we hear the very real fact that men can suffer a reduction in libido after childbirth, too.

A shift happens for many men once a baby has come out of their lover's body. This shift is generally psychological more than physical. While every woman who carries a child experiences a weakened pelvic floor, the difference is not as profound as you

might imagine. Looser vaginal muscles gradually snap back into shape and the body returns to its former state, especially if you practice your Kegel exercises (for more on how to do this, see page 103). What is sometimes more difficult to change is your partner's struggle to view the mother of his children in the same sexy light he did before your roles changed and you became co-parents as well as lovers.

The most important thing is to plan for these changes and anticipate that your new roles as parents will impact your sex life and your unique connection. In fact, before the baby comes, you might want to prepare by discussing your expectations and planning how you expect your relationship and your time together to change.

Fortunately, for many couples, parenthood can and should increase their bond, and may even help decrease inhibitions in the bedroom. However, like any major relationship change, working your way to that point will take clear communication, honesty, and a little bit of hard work.

The truth about...

DEALING WITH INFERTILITY

It is estimated that one in every eight childbearing couples struggle with infertility issues. This adds emotional strain to a couple's relationship, and also complicates the sexual bond. In order to keep your relationship on track under these challenging circumstances, try to think of sex as more than just "baby-making." Consider having "baby-making sex" in one room or in one position, and then having "relationship sex" in other places or positions. This will keep part of your sex life fun and pressure free.

TOP 5

WAYS TO KEEP KIDS FROM RUINING YOUR SEX LIFE

Kids are a delight, but they can also be problematic when it comes to keeping the spark alive in your relationship. In today's child-centric society, it can be difficult to find couple time, which means that it can be difficult to feel romantic toward your partner. If you want your relationship to last and be fulfilling, you must stop putting the kids before your relationship. It is only when you put each other above everyone else that you can truly find the intimacy and passion you crave.

1 Embrace separate beds.
It might be hard to turn away the kiddies, especially when they are so fun to cuddle, but cuddling your partner is equally vital. More importantly, your kids need to learn how to sleep alone and be independent. It may be hard to get them into their own beds, but if you are consistent they'll ultimately make the transition and you'll get back those stolen moments in bed.

2 Distinguish between vacations and family trips and take both.
While it is wonderful to see your child experience the beach or Disneyland for the first time, this type of trip does not give you the mental and physical break you need. Remember to budget time and money for adult-only vacations in which you can get away with your spouse solo and really reconnect.

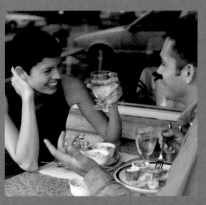

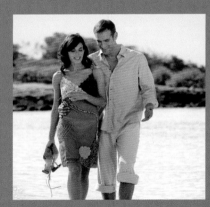

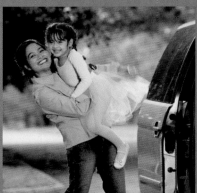

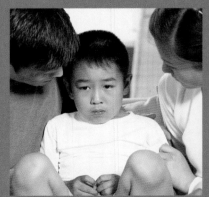

3 Don't try to be a superparent.

Limit your children's after-school activities to just one or two each season. If you run yourself ragged driving your children to every activity under the sun, you won't have time or energy for romance or sex. Remember, too, to take advantage of scheduled activities: An empty house means valuable private time for you and your partner.

4 Set a united front.

When your children try to get a "yes" out of Mommy after Daddy has already said "no," your connection can suffer. If one of you feels as though your opinion has been disregarded, it can be very hard to turn off that frustration and get in the mood. Bypass these issues by agreeing to never disagree about discipline in front of the kids.

5 Write date night in stone—always.

Most couples love date night, yet it often gets pushed aside due to little family disturbances. Set your time together in stone, even if little Jimmy really wants to have friends over. Couples must have alone time together in which they can bond and be intimate, so date night should only be canceled for truly unavoidable conflicts.

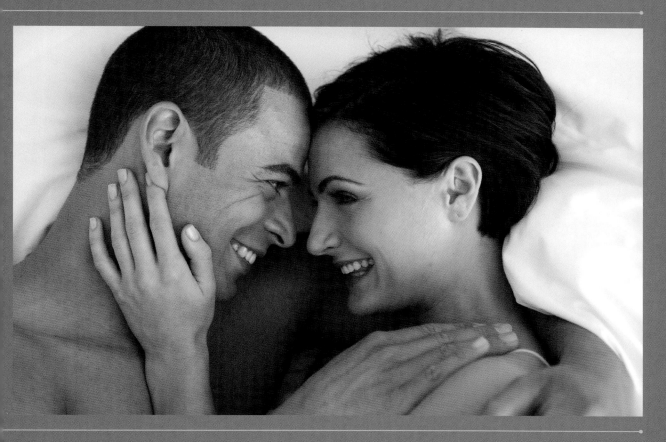

The new date night

Remember when you were getting ready to go out on a date with someone you really liked? All those feeling of butterflies and anticipation don't have to disappear in a long-term relationship. In fact, it can be easier than you think to get back some of that old feeling. You just have to step out of your routine—and perhaps a little out of your comfort zone.

Creative dating

More often than not, your dating life falls to the bottom of the list when life runs you ragged. There are tons of excuses, from being too tired to being short on cash, but just like everything else in life, you can solve these problems with a little creativity. You don't have to spend a lot of money to go on a date—you don't even have to leave the house. Whether it's setting up a picnic in your living room or cooking a new cuisine together, date night can be as sexy and silly and inexpensive as you want it to be. In fact, the sexier and sillier your dates are, the better. Letting date night become a dull night because you do the same thing every time you go out (dinner? movie?), will cause your enjoyment of the night and each other to suffer.

The surrender date

A great way to liven up date night is what I call a "surrender date." It's easy and fun, particularly for the type A women and control freaks out there. A surrender date requires that you give up control and sit back and relax. The gist of it is this: Your partner agrees to do all of the planning, and you agree to go along for the ride. In order for it to work, each of you really has to hold up your end of the bargain.

First and perhaps most important, the surrender date planner does everything from start to finish. He picks out your clothes and jewelry (and even your underwear!), decides when and where you're going, and takes charge of all the logistics, such as transportation and money. The first time you go on a surrender date, it may feel a little too scary to give up all that control—but that's the point. A surrender date isn't just some kitschy idea that you'll be bored with in five minutes. It really shakes up your routine and your relationship. A little bit of pressure helps to inspire creativity in your partner and a stronger sense of trust in you.

As for what to do, the options are endless. You may choose to relive a past date or try a new adventure. You can challenge yourself to try something new, like taking tennis lessons or joining a salsa class, or seek out comedy clubs or blues joints that you might not have considered before. The more adventurous your dating life, the more excited and intimate you will be as a couple.

In addition, giving up control can be incredibly exhilarating, which is something that few women think about. Putting timeworn activities and roles to rest is a good thing. Surrender dates introduce new sensations and pleasures to your love life, which is a necessary part of keeping your spark alive.

The truth about...

DATING ON A BUDGET

Inexpensive dates can turn into some of your best memories. Sign up for a free cooking class at a local restaurant or kitchen supply store; roast s'mores and set up a tent in your backyard; go to a drive-in movie and bring your own snacks. Try it and you'll see: There truly are endless options to have fun together without spending a great deal of money.

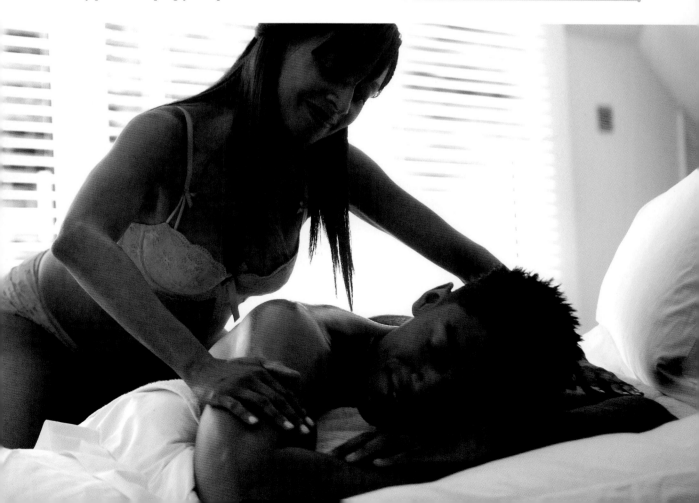

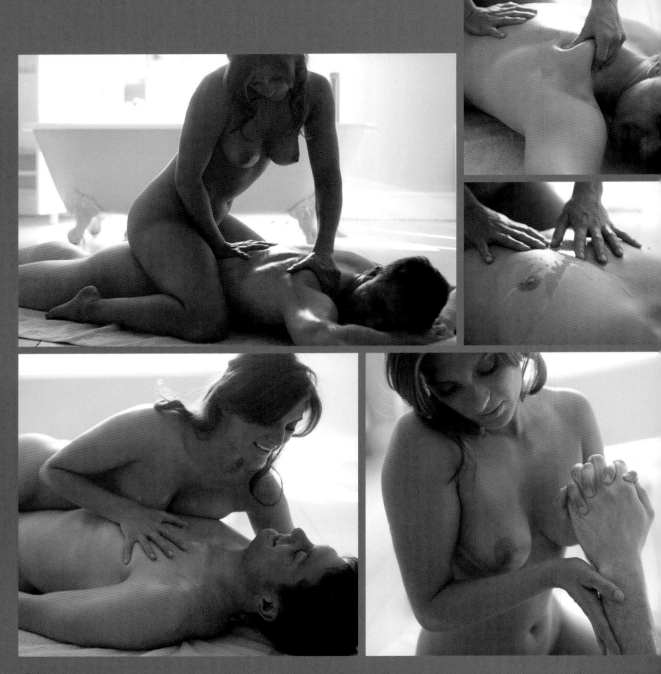

Oil up

A massage can be one of the most sensual and bonding parts of foreplay. The trick to maximizing eroticism is to focus on the way your partner's body responds. Notice when his muscles relax, how he breathes, when he sighs in pleasure. Move slowly, lingering over every erogenous zone and enjoying the sensation of his skin. Touching like this will make you both a better masseuse and a better lover.

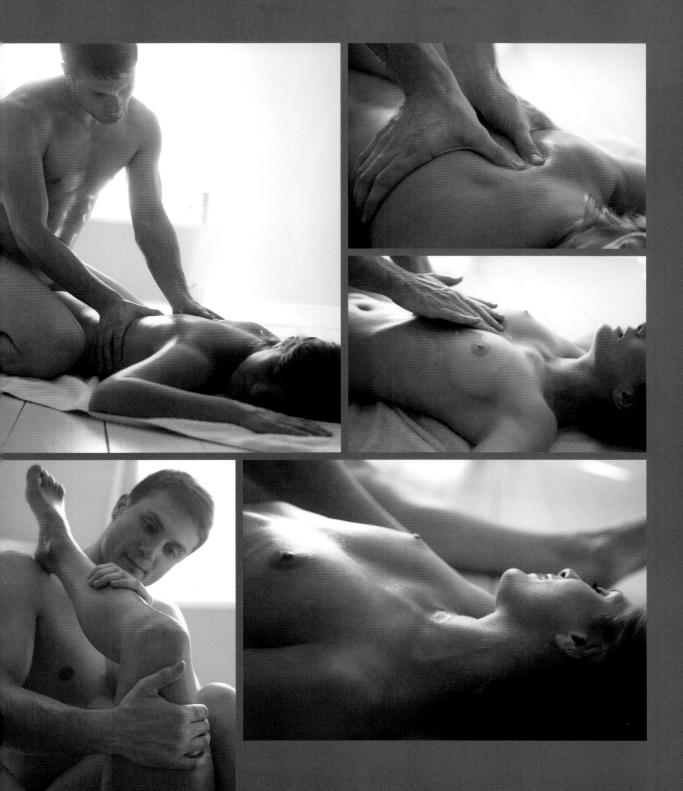

The importance of girlfriends

Maintaining your friendships can actually be one of the best ways to also maintain your relationship. This is true even though it means that you may spend more time apart from your significant other. The reason? Spending time with other women helps you relax, refresh, and remember all the things you love about yourself as a woman—which in turn gives you potent feminine energy to bring to your relationship.

The instant stress-reliever

How do you relax after a bad day at work? What do you do to calm down after a fight with your spouse? Your response will probably depend on your gender. When men are under stress, the hormones in their bodies prompt the "fight-or-flight" response. This response was very important for our male ancestors, as it helped them to either fight off or flee from danger. In the cavemen era, this meant attacking the wild animal or running for dear life. In our modern era, it might mean getting into a shouting match, or shutting down completely and seething alone for a while when confronted with a stressful situation.

For years, researchers assumed that both men and women processed stress chemicals in the same manner. However, recent studies have found that when women are under stress, they may experience a different reaction: the tend-and-befriend response. This response also harkens back to the cavemen days. While it may have benefited men to run or to fight when confronted with danger, women—who were at home caring for the young members of the tribe—had to protect their children (tend) and rely on other women for support (befriend).

Centuries later, these ancient models for behavior may still exist. When most men have a bad day they simply want to go home and forget the situation (a flight response). Women, on the other hand, generally want to call a girlfriend or female family member to vent and analyze the situation (a befriend response). At one time, this female bonding and sharing of information may have helped women survive potentially dangerous situations, so it is no wonder that women often feel like chatting with a friend when they are stressed or anxious. Both the male and female responses are natural and fitting, and neither partner will derive the same amount of comfort if they are not allowed the type of stress release that they crave.

Protecting your friendships

Despite this, many women find that female friendship falls by the wayside in the face of career, marriage, kids, and other responsibilities. This loss of female friendship is devastating. The connections women have with each other are powerful and ancestral, and without them, we lose a crucial part of ourselves.

Making time for your girlfriends is a quick way to get an energy and mood boost. Many studies have found that friendships are crucial not only for our emotional health, but also for our physical health. When you make time for your girlfriends, you make time for fun and laughter, but you also gain something deeper. The energy, empathy, support, and encouragement that you receive from each other during this male-free time is like a shot of energy to your psyche. Spending time with other women can help decrease stress and enhance oxytocin, which has a calming effect on the brain. In fact, it seems that when the hormone oxytocin is released as part of a woman's stress response, it buffers the fight-or-flight response and encourages her to tend children and gather with other women. When she engages in this tending or befriending, studies suggest that more oxytocin is released, further countering stress.

To maximize your time for friendship, remember that you don't have to choose frivolous activities. You can volunteer together, or train for a marathon. The most important benefit is that spending time with other women will allow you to simply be yourself, rather than being attached to the persona of mother or wife. There is an energy we gain from other women that cannot come from anywhere else. No matter how much love we have for our children and our partners, nothing can replace the connection we share with female friends. So, call your friends and reconnect. Plan a trip, big or small. Just don't forget, you never outgrow your need for friends!

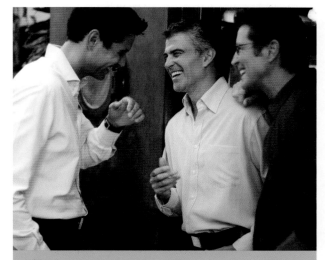

The truth about...

MALE FRIENDSHIPS

A UCLA study found that while estrogen can enhance oxytocin and thus ease stress in women, a similar calming response does not occur in men. This is because while estrogen promotes oxytocin, testosterone—which men produce in high levels when they're under stress—seems to reduce this effect. Perhaps this explains why spending time with your girlfriends is so important to you, while your partner can go weeks without calling his buddies.

However, it's equally important that your partner stays connected to who he was before your relationship began. Neither of you should abandon your old interests or friendships. Hanging out with his friends will give your partner a valuable sense of independence, and time to relax. Spending time apart helps you to remain multifaceted, interesting people to each other and to the outside world. This is just one of the reasons that friendships are so crucial.

Getting along with your in-laws

No family is picture-perfect. From feuding in-laws to antagonistic family friends, every relationship comes with its share of baggage. Understanding your partner's difficult mother, or helping him grasp your brother's sarcastic sense of humor, is all part of being in a long-term relationship. When you take the time to do this, you will not only strengthen your relationship with your partner, you will also help make family gatherings less stressful.

Making family time a part of life

If the only time you ever see your in-laws is during the hectic holiday season, it is no wonder that you find yourself particularly sensitive or edgy when they are around. In contrast, if you build up an ongoing relationship with them, it will be that much easier to understand your in-laws and appreciate the nicer things about them. It will also help create more ease in your relationship. I have found that in-laws are most difficult when they feel shut out of your lives. When they feel involved, they are more likely to support your choices as a family.

Nevertheless, if in-laws are often difficult or disrespectful, it is natural to want to avoid spending time with them. Remember, however, that fighting to love applies to your family as well. If you can fight for your family's well-being, happiness, and success instead of your own desire to be right, you will drastically eliminate the stress in this relationship. Part of fighting to love means reaching out to your in-laws and helping them feel included and welcome in your life as a family. The more often you do this, the more likely it is that their defenses will go down and they will be less critical.

Accepting your family

Although we want the people in our lives to be kind and charming, the truth is that sometimes people are difficult or even toxic. A toxic person routinely makes you feel badly about yourself, or attacks you and your loved ones. You may not be able to avoid these situations, but you can take control of how it affects your emotional health by learning to accept your relative's shortcomings and set boundaries.

In the beginning, accepting your relative's imperfections can be hard. Maybe you always imagined that you and your mother would be best friends when you grew up, or that your father would be a mentor for your husband. But then, reality kicked in—you and your mother still argue, and your partner and father have different interests and personalities. Rather than fighting life's realities, try to find beauty in the imperfections. Maybe your mother is brusque, but she has a great sense of humor. Maybe your partner doesn't get along with your father, but he does click with your uncle. Do what you can to make family relationships work, and then step back and let people take responsibility for their own behavior.

It is also a good idea to set family boundaries. This requires that you are open and direct about your feelings. For example, if your mother-in-law insults your cooking, be honest with her about how it makes you feel. By setting boundaries, you can help make your needs clear to those around you. You will also feel better simply by getting things off your chest.

Once you make your boundaries known, it is up to the other person to change the behavior. If he or she is incapable or unwilling, you will have to make a decision. You can either separate yourself from that person as much as possible, or try to ignore the behavior whenever you do come into contact with each other. Either option will be difficult. Cutting a relative out of your life (even a toxic relative) can be very upsetting and scary, but it might ultimately be the best decision for you and your family. You have the right to decide who gets to be in your life, and if you have done everything you can to work out the relationship, your partner should support your decision, even if the person in question is his relative. Sometimes distance is necessary in order to encourage a toxic relative to change and reconcile.

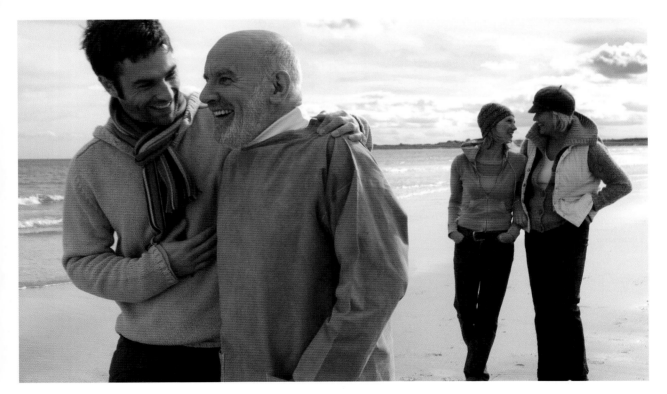

The sandwich generation

Whether your parents live with you or somewhere else, many women now find themselves in the middle, juggling the needs of older parents, while caring for young children at the same time. This phenomenon is known as the "sandwich generation" and more and more women are finding themselves in the eye of the storm, trying to keep everyone happy and healthy, with very little time to take care of their own personal needs.

The caregiver role

Thanks to modern medicine, people are living longer than ever before. However, seniors often need additional help and care, and most families either can't afford it, or hate the thought of sending their loved one to a nursing home. Instead, more families than ever are opting to open up their homes and adopt the older generation. While this is a lovely way to serve the parents who once took care of you, it does add to your list of responsibilities and can be a strain on your relationship.

Caregiver burnout is a very real concern for these overscheduled and overstressed women and men. Not only do caregivers have a million things on their to-do lists, but they also have to deal with the emotions that stem from seeing a parent losing his or her physical or mental capabilities. This is often a scary and lonely time, and it causes many people to clam up and simply focus on the physical tasks they can control, such as sweeping the floor or tackling the laundry, rather than talking to their partner or reconnecting over dinner with a friend.

The most important thing to remember during this time is that you need help and you can't do it all by yourself. Trying to do it all is never the answer (for more on this, see pages 26–27 on the costs of **Hero** behavior). In fact, it's the surest way to caregiver burnout, and will not only take a toll on your own quality of life, but on you relationship and your family, too. I know it's tempting to try to push through it, imagining a potential light at the end of the tunnel that you can't yet see, but it doesn't work that way. The tunnel gets longer for a million different reasons: when you get sick, when you lose your temper, or when you start to lose your way in your most important relationships because of the stress. The sooner you start asking for help, the sooner you can focus some of your attention on keeping yourself strong. Remember that it isn't

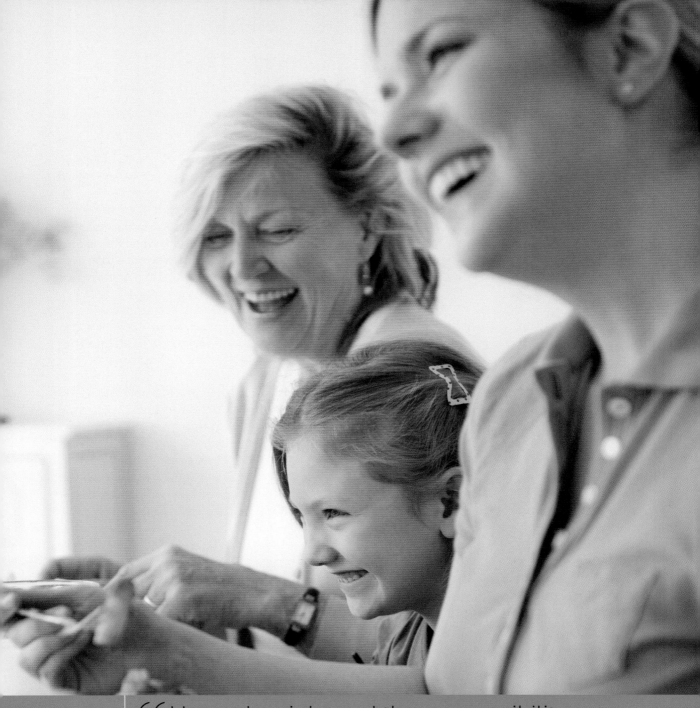

66 I have the right and the responsibility to make time for myself so that I can relax. 99

> **❝**Finding moments of relaxation will help you build the reservoir of energy to be a better caregiver.**❞**

abandoning those you love when you take a break to do something special for yourself. It is only by finding those moments of relaxation that you can build the reservoir of energy that will make you a better partner and caregiver. Stepping away from self-blame and realizing that the world won't end if you release control is crucial for your health.

There are many resources for caregivers out there, including online forums, support groups, and books (for more on this, see Resources, page 251). In addition, support can likely be found among friends and family. When you get over any embarrassment or guilt you feel over asking for help, you'll find many around you who will step up and offer support.

There are likely a number of resources in your community, as well, which can help to lighten your load. Look for a caregiver you can hire to come look after your parent while you shop for groceries, or consider signing up for a food delivery service that will shorten your to-do list. Hospice is also an amazing resource if someone you love has been diagnosed with a terminal illness, even if they are not very sick. Investigate the hospice centers in your community—most will come to your home and watch over your parent or relative, which can give you a few hours to take for yourself, or even a few days in which you and your partner can get away for some much-needed R&R.

Maintaining your relationship

Finding time for your relationship and your sex life won't always be easy. It is very hard to feel sexually desirable and in tune with your partner when you are lacking the time, energy, and motivation to be

sexual. However, the benefits of intimacy can go a long way toward helping you feel happier and healthier. Sex can release endorphins and reduce stress, and will keep you connected with your partner. Thus, rather than thinking of sex as a chore, think of it as a way to take care of yourself. Even if your motivation is lacking and you find yourself "just doing it," you will still reap the benefits of renewed intimacy. (See page 151 for more on the "just do it" philosophy.)

Protecting your emotional health

It is also important to care for your own emotional health during this time, particularly when you are struggling with feelings of sadness or even guilt. Oftentimes, people feel guilty or helpless when a parent or close family member becomes sick. They wonder if they are allowed to be happy or have fun while someone who is so important to them is unwell. Even if your parent isn't living with you, there can still be a tremendous amount of pressure to do everything in your power to care for him or her, including managing the finances, cooking, cleaning the house, managing medical care—the list goes on and on. With so much to do, it can be hard to put yourself first, or even put your personal needs on your to-do list at all. However, remember that no matter how sick or needy your parents may be, they want you to be happy (for more on this, see page 16 on self-blame and how to recover from it).

If you aren't in good health and good spirits, you won't be able to help those around you to the extent that you wish. You also won't be able to be present with those you love, or stay positive in your daily life and relationships. Putting yourself first means honoring your needs so that you can move forward to care for those around you efficiently and in a way that works for you and the ones you love.

It's also important to remember that this is a difficult time for your whole family, not just for you. Everyone is going to be a little on edge, including your partner. In fact, men might even be more at risk of suffering from caregiver burnout, because they are less likely to open up and talk about their feelings, and they want to be strong for their families during this difficult time. Encouraging your partner to make time for himself and express his feelings is important. Let him know that it is okay to be sad or scared, or even to feel helpless at times. Remind him that you don't need him to know all the answers, you just need his love and support. Sickness is a situation you cannot control, and trying to do this will only stress you out.

Your children also might resent the attention they have lost, and may act out to win back the spotlight. Ultimately, everyone is going to need some time to adjust and find their footing once family dynamics change. However, with communication, love, and openness, you can make this a truly rewarding and life-affirming experience.

Expressing your emotions

Along with reaching out for help and taking care of yourself, it's crucial to communicate to your partner your feeling about what is going on in your home. It's okay to voice things like "I feel so overwhelmed. I don't know if I can do this" or "Sometimes I wish it could be like it was before my father was sick." You aren't a bad person if you secretly wish that you didn't have to take care of your parent, or that you could have your free time back. It's only human to feel this way, just like it's only human to also feel scared, hurt, angry, and depressed during challenging times. A therapist can help you work through these feelings if they become overwhelming.

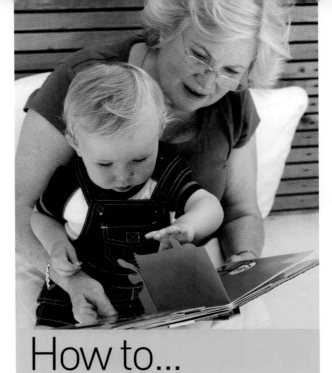

How to...

FIND TIME FOR YOUR PARTNER

In order to make time for your relationship, it's important to get creative—and to get the whole family involved in protecting and facilitating your time alone as a couple. This time will help you both maintain the energy to be the rock of support your family needs. Here's one way to do this.

1 If a live-in relative is able, have him or her help out with small household tasks, or ask that he or she take care of your children for a few hours. This not only takes some things off your plate, it helps give your parent a sense of purpose and pride.

2 Need suggestions? Simple activities like reading a book or baking pre-made cookie dough will be fun for both your parent and your child, and won't be too strenuous if your parent is low on energy.

3 Meanwhile, you can enjoy some quality time with your husband. Take a short, sensual break for a picnic of wine and cheese in the backyard or a romantic, soothing bubble bath.

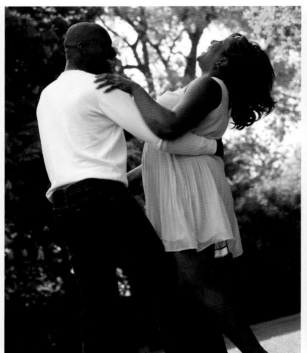
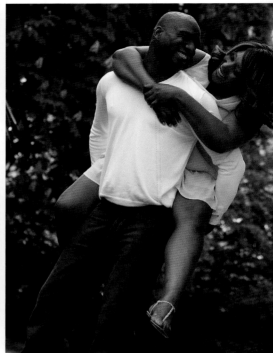

Chapter 9

Making the life you want

Recognizing that you can choose to be happy in every area of your life is an absolutely revolutionary truth. It can entirely change your perspective on your past, your plans for your future, and the way you presently experience your relationship. Learning to embrace honesty and authenticity, and to do away with time-consuming trivialities, will help you create the life you truly want.

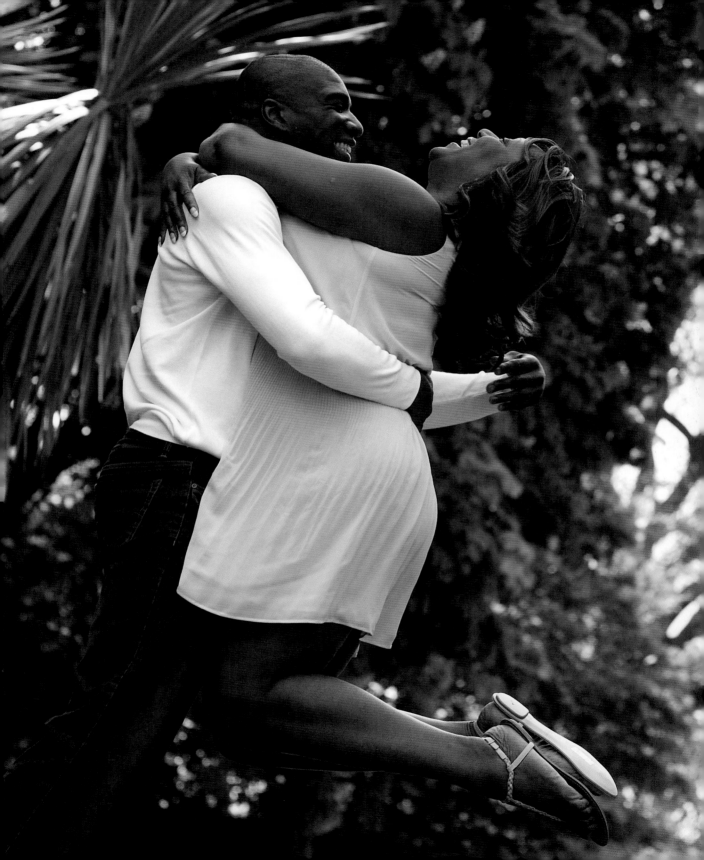

How often do you choose to be happy in your life and relationship? This is a question that few of us stop to ask ourselves. Popular culture trains us to think that happiness simply happens for certain people, when the reality is that we truly can control how happy we are. Think honestly about these questions, evaluating how you respond to the everyday scenarios that impact our relationships. More than big life changes, it is these situations that often determine whether we are happy, or frustrated and unfulfilled.

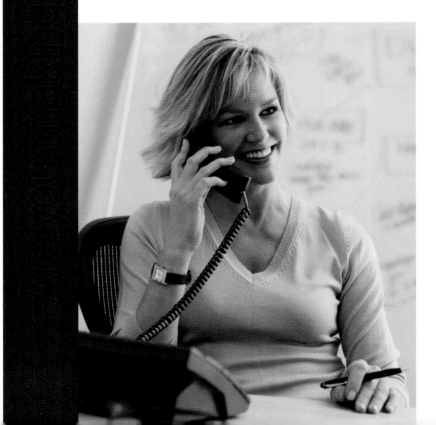

1 YOUR CURRENT JOB IS FAR FROM THE JOB OF YOUR dreams. You know that you need to make a change in order to get into the right career path, so you:

A Have every intention to start looking for new jobs, but can only find time to complain often about how much you hate your job. If only your life had turned out more like you planned!

B Quit your job and decide to take a break for a while. When the job market opens up, you will begin searching and try to land a better job.

C Make a commitment to apply to 10 new jobs each week, and continue to invest time and energy in your current job in the meantime. The better referrals you can give, the more likely you are to land the job you want.

2 YOU HAVEN'T HAD MUCH TIME TO SEE YOUR FRIENDS lately, because you are juggling so many work and family commitments. When a chance arises to get away for an impromptu girls' weekend at your friend's nearby lake house, you:

A Pass on the opportunity. As much as you miss your girlfriends, you don't feel like you have time or money to spend away from your family right now.

B Tell your friends that you can only go if you do it on your time schedule (two months from now). It's not your fault you are busier than they are!

C Ask your partner if it's okay with him if you jet away for two days of girlfriend time, promising to repay the favor the next time his golfing buddies make plans to get together. You both need this time with friends.

3 YOU WANT TO SETTLE DOWN AND FOCUS ON

raising a family, but your partner isn't ready to have children yet. You:

Ⓐ Complain about his resistance to have children to your friends, sister, and coworkers. He is being totally unreasonable and selfish.

Ⓑ Feel angry and suspicious. If he isn't committed enough to have children with you, then maybe he simply isn't committed.

Ⓒ Sit down and talk with him about your feelings so that you can work out a compromise, such as trying to have children in a year's time. You don't want to rush something so important.

4 SINCE YOU GAVE BIRTH TWO YEARS AGO,

you have been miserable about your weight gain. Deciding it is time to do something about it, you:

Ⓐ Go on a new diet. Who knows? This time it may be a plan that will inspire your willpower to kick in.

Ⓑ Try to accept it for the time being, hoping that your body image will improve and that you will feel more comfortable being sexual with your partner over time.

Ⓒ Forget the diet plans and focus more on getting healthy, committing to cutting out unhealthy foods and exercising a few times a week with several of your friends.

5 YOU WANT TO IMPROVE YOUR RELATIONSHIP AND

have a fulfilling, fun marriage. In order to achieve this, you:

Ⓐ Try to convince your partner to watch a lot of romantic comedies. Maybe then he'll be inspired to take you on a hot air balloon ride or plan the exotic vacation of your dreams.

Ⓑ Have a talk with him and explain that he just isn't spontaneous or romantic enough, and that he needs to change in order for you to be happy.

Ⓒ Plan a special dinner for him in hopes of showing him that romance is important for your relationship, and inspiring him to think about what feels romantic to you.

6 YOU'VE HAD A LONG, DRAINING DAY AT WORK.

As soon as you get home, you:

Ⓐ Curl up on the couch with your latest romance novel and a pint of ice cream. Escaping from reality always makes you feel better.

Ⓑ Start an argument with your partner over who is going to get dinner ready despite your best intentions to put your bad day behind you. He is just so unhelpful sometimes!

Ⓒ Pour a glass of wine, turn on some relaxing music, and chat with your partner while he cooks for you, promising him that you'll do the dishes after dinner.

A-type answers suggest that you may be stuck in the **Victim** role (for more on this type of behavior, see page 24). **Victims** aren't proactive, and don't recognize their own power in most situations. Because of this, they often blame others for their own unhappiness. You are likely acting passive and unhappy, watching your own life go by without any sense of control.

B-type answers mean that you may be stuck in the **Villain** role (for more on this type of behavior, see page 26). You tend to vocally blame your partner or those around you for your own unhappiness, and it is often hard for you to take responsibility for what's not working in your life. Instead, you accuse others of creating problems, and are unable to relax or be happy.

C-type answers indicate that you are generally proactive when it comes to improving your life situation, and are empowered to make the changes that get you where you want to go. Congratulations! You truly are choosing happiness.

❝ The way we respond to small, everyday situations often determines whether we are happy or unfulfilled. ❞

Choosing happiness

What's the secret to a happy life and a loving relationship? Some people think the secret is money, others think it's success, and still others think the answer lies in physical "perfection" or the proverbial house and white picket fence. But the real secret is that you choose to create happiness for yourself.

Dwelling in joy

All of the things listed above can bring you temporary joy, but as philosophers and leaders of every religion have told us, the only secret to happiness is accepting, finding, and embracing the joy that already exists in and around you. Any journey we take to find happiness will ultimately be unfulfilling unless it leads us back to the original truth—that we already have everything we need to be happy.

Leading a life of joy isn't easy, yet it is the goal of everyone on this planet. We all want peaceful relationships and fulfilling love lives, yet we constantly stand in our own way. We find little flaws in our partner or reasons why our relationship isn't working. Then, instead of taking action to create the life we want, we sit around and mope or engage in harmful coping behaviors, whether that's drinking too much, forgoing exercise and eating junk food, or playing the blame game with our partner, coworkers, or loved ones.

My inspiration for writing this book was to empower you to jump off the bandwagon of blame and learn how to let go of useless, self-sabotaging behaviors like complaining or self-pity. This isn't to say that difficult times or even tragedies won't come along, or that your partner is always going to be perfect. Sometimes it will be very hard not to complain. Sometimes your partner will be completely wrong or even selfish—and sometimes you will be, too. However, by learning to accept the inevitability of life's imperfections, you can still move forward and reach your goal of creating the life you want. It all starts and ends with you. Only you can do it.

Your dream relationship

As illustrated throughout this book, creating the relationship of your dreams starts with becoming the best version of yourself. Rather than looking for someone to complete you or someone to fix you (or for someone who you can fix), it's time to put your focus on finding happiness within yourself. Changes that we've discussed, like learning to communicate authentically, empowering yourself to take charge of your life and your health, and learning how to stop the blame game, are all part of this process. They are small changes, but they are crucial to your relationship health and happiness.

Every relationship takes work and plenty of effort. Even the most well-matched couple will encounter bumps in the road and ebbs and flows in their relationship. Learning how to circumvent these problems and grow within the relationship is a crucial part of finding, developing, and keeping the love you want. Blame can't have any role in a happy relationship, or in a happy life.

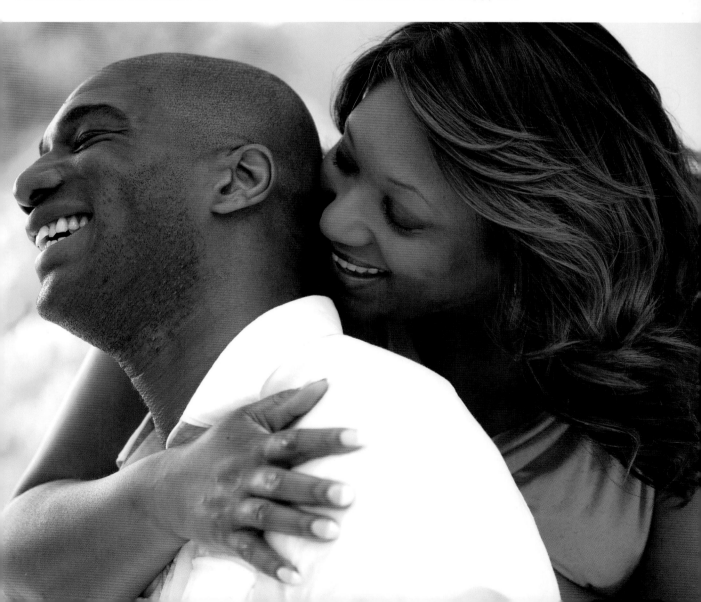

Practicing authenticity

Communicating authentically can be very hard to do, but the rewards are great. When you are honest with yourself about your true feelings, the areas where you feel "stuck" or trapped by emotion, and the personas that are an integral part of your personality, you will lessen the power that any negative emotion has in your life. You will then be able to build a life—and a relationship—that is more loving and real.

Moving your feelings

Remember, there are only five real feelings: joy, sadness, anger, fear, and sexual attraction. Every other feeling is an incarnation of one of these. So, whenever you feel stuck in an emotion, take a step back and identify which core feeling you are experiencing. Once identified, go ahead and really feel it, whether it means crying or screaming into a sink full of water or punching a pillow. A really authentic feeling only takes about 20–30 seconds to move through you if you let it run its course.

Sometimes you may let yourself cry or scream or otherwise try to move your feelings, and you won't start feeling better. If you still feel mistreated and angry, you are probably stuck in a persona. Until you move out of that persona, you won't be able to shift your mood in the way that you want.

Living with your personas

We all have a number of different personas (for more on common types of personas, see pages 48–51). Each persona has value and serves or has served you in some way, even the so-called negative ones. For example, maybe your "Polly Pleaser" persona was the key to getting through your childhood with an alcoholic or abandoning parent. As long as you were a good girl, you wouldn't attract any negative attention. Understanding our personas can teach us valuable lessons about ourselves, so don't be ashamed or embarrassed of them. The same is true for your partner's personas. Learning to love and accept these very specific roles you fall into will go a long way in helping you shift and begin communicating clearly and authentically.

Personas are like an array of different coats. What you want is to choose to put that coat on rather than having it stuck onto you against your wishes. To do this, a good first step is to name your persona. Are you a Grumpy Griper? A Drama Queen Delilah?

Make up a name that resonates with you and will help you connect with your persona when you are wearing it against your will. For example, I have a persona called "Dire Mama" who thinks everything with my children is life or death. I can absolutely love and appreciate the essence of Dire Mama. She's the one who makes sure the kids eat healthily, are socially responsible, and know how to be a friend. She serves me and those around me, but sometimes I get stuck in that persona and that's not fun or helpful for my family or for me.

When this happens, the quickest fix is to have some fun. Exaggerate your persona and act her out, blowing her out of proportion in an entertaining way. For example, if you are stuck in a drama queen role, play it up and fling yourself around the room with the back of your hand on your forehead. I do this with my kids all the time. Sometimes when Dire

Mama has a grip on me and I'm acting tense and angry, I gasp and spell out an exaggerated path of concern. I might shriek, "Oh my goodness! This is horrible! You are watching more than an hour of TV! Your brain will turn to mush and you'll melt into the ground! You won't go to college! You won't have a job! This is horrible! Terrible!" The kids think it's hilarious and often play along and interact with Dire Mama. They sometimes even say to me, "Um, Mommy? I think you need to shift!"

When your kids or partner become your allies and help you play out a persona, it can then lose its grip on you. By recognizing when you are stuck, identifying the feeling underneath it, moving out of your persona, and allowing emotions to pass, you will be able to shift and create a more authentic life—and more authentic relationships. Processing your emotions in this way leads to empowerment and peace.

Making a physical shift

Diana Chapman, a respected life coach, has shared with me some wonderful ideas for shifting from her "shift deck." Let me warn you in advance that they sound silly—but they really work. In fact, being silly is part of the point. It's hard to be stuck in a negative mood when you start getting playful.

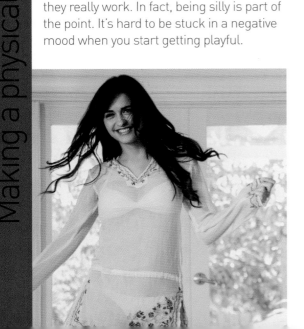

Express your feelings

- **Complain about your issue,** finishing each sentence with " . . . and I'm sexy."
- **Make a puppet with your hand** and have your puppet talk about your issue.
- **Describe in detail a sensation** that you are feeling in your body right now.
- **While wiggling your butt,** repeat and finish this sentence at least three times "What I really want is . . . "

It may seem ridiculous at first, but it works. Moving your body in crazy ways or acting out funny scenarios is a sure-fire way to take your mind off whatever is bothering you and to help release any built-up tension or stress. As Diana often says, "the only thing more fun than drama is play." (For more ideas on how to shift, see pages 18–19.)

Embracing honesty

In order to create the life you want, you know that you have to create the communication that supports it. You might have mastered all the communication techniques in this book. However, there is still one important lesson left to learn: the importance of being authentic and letting go of the urge to tell all those little white lies and tiny mistruths.

The little white lie

Many people believe that they are truthful with their significant others, but recent studies have shown that people tell white lies by the dozen each day. Consider how many little lies you have told your lover lately. Did you pretend to like his hideous shirt? Did you act as though you loved her dry turkey pot pie? Did you falsely assure him that those extra five pounds weren't noticeable?

If so, don't feel guilty—you are not alone. Nearly everyone tells white lies in order to protect other people's feelings or avoid conflict. In fact, a recent study, found that children as young as three years old were capable of white lies. Parents often teach their children that "honesty is the best policy," but they don't necessarily model that in their own lives. Our kids watch us make up excuses to skip out of a party we don't want to attend, or they see us being overly friendly to an acquaintance we bad-mouth in private. We want our children to fake enthusiasm and pleasure upon receiving a horrible gift from Grandma, and they soon learn to use white lies in other situations as well. It is a natural human inclination, but not one that always serves to build strong, trust-filled relationships.

White lies in relationships

In a relationship, any lie or withholding of the truth, no matter how innocent, can keep you and your partner from having the openness and intimacy you crave. This is especially true in sexual relationships. Many women pretend to enjoy their humdrum sexual experiences, even going so far as to fake orgasm. In fact, some women go their entire lives never owning up to their sexual discontent, merely because they do not want to hurt their partner's feelings. If this type of sexual pretense resonates with you, the important thing to remember is that most men crave feedback on their sexual performance—and not necessarily of the generic "Baby, you were great" variety. Men need specifics, both when they are doing something right and when they are doing something wrong. If you don't tell your partner about your sexual experience, there is no real way for him to figure out what you're thinking and feeling.

General white lies can also impact your relationship, even if they don't directly relate to your sex life. White lies build up over time and take away a piece of your authentic being each time you voice them. The momentary comfort these lies provide is truly not worth the toll they ultimately take on your relationship. Yes, it is scary to be honest, but if you can do so in a loving and positive way, it is immeasurably better for your relationship. You may intend for your little mistruths to make other people feel better, but this is not a good idea if it's at the expense of your own happiness, your partner's happiness, or your closeness as a couple.

Committing to truth

A wise pact to make is to agree with your partner that you are going to tell him the truth, even if it's not always positive. If you talk openly about this agreement then you will both know what to expect, and honest feedback will be less likely to come as a shock. Sometimes the white lie seems like the easy way out, but what may seem easier in the short term often comes back to haunt you in the long term. Once you get into the habit of being honest with your spouse, you will find that your level of trust grows and that both of your ability to accept negative feedback grows, as well.

That doesn't mean that you have to always speak the harsh truth. For instance, if your partner asks if you notice those five pounds he's gained, you can say: "You look handsome no matter what, honey, and if you want to lose weight I'll work out

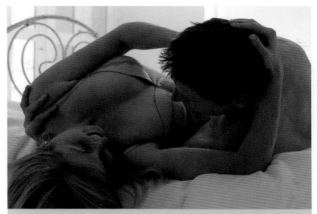

How to...

GIVE YOUR PARTNER HONEST BEDROOM FEEDBACK

Men want honesty, yes, but make sure that your tone is neither critical nor bitter. Understandably, this is a sensitive topic. You can help prevent hurting your partner's feelings by saving any less-than-positive feedback for outside the bedroom, when his vulnerabilities aren't so high. Here's how to be completely honest in the bedroom.

1 Try couching your suggestion inside a compliment, such as: "Honey, I love it when you kiss me slowly, especially during foreplay."

2 When he does something you like in the bedroom, be sure to coo or moan your approval.

3 When he does something you don't like, it's important to be a little more gentle and discreet with your feedback, especially if it's in the moment. Try shifting positions ever so slightly or moving his hand to a more erogenous spot.

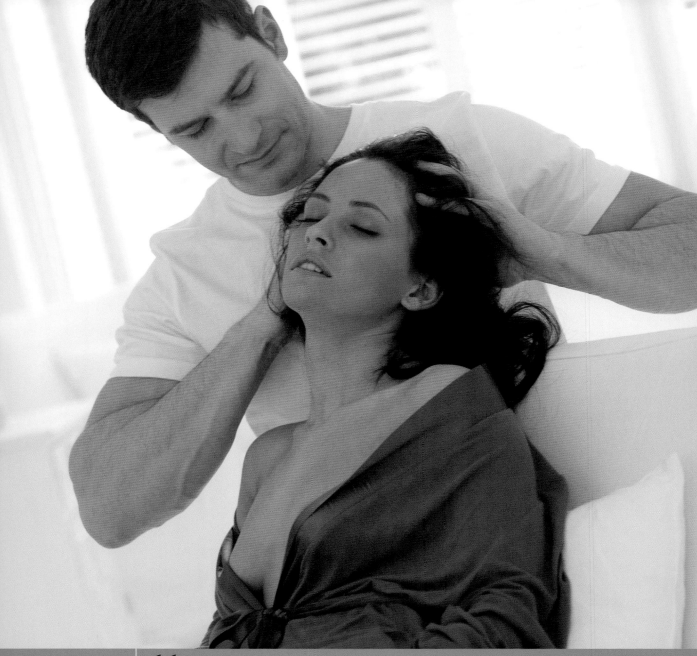

66 I will share my fantasies, but will make sure
they don't harm the reality of our relationship. **99**

with you and help in any way I can." Or, instead of agreeing that the evening with his parents was a fantastic time, talk about the things you appreciated about the evening, but be gently honest about the parts that were uncomfortable. For example, you might say: "Your mother is a great cook, but I have to be honest and say I was hurt by the comment she made about the way we raise the kids."

The bottom line is that there is no replacement for honesty in a relationship, sexually or otherwise. Great sex and great communication take work—they are never as simple as they look in the movies. Being completely honest with each other can work wonders in your relationship. You will experience a new sense of openness and won't feel those nagging, unspoken tensions between you. Even better, you will no longer feel compelled to hide your true feelings or insecurities from your partner.

Saying too much

There are really only two ways that being too open can lead to relationship trouble. Both of these occur in the sexual realm. First, I'm a big proponent of sharing your sexual fantasies with your partner. It's a great way to open up to each other and choose to experiment more in the bedroom. However, when that fantasy is about a real person in your life—your neighbor, your partner's brother, your daughter's soccer coach—I don't suggest telling your partner about it. This will only lead to insecurity, and is simply not necessary to share, unless you are really longing to act it out in real life. At that point, it's important to honestly address what's not working in your relationship, ideally with the help of a therapist (for more on how to do this, see pages 76–77). In any other case, sharing this fantasy makes it more of a reality than it really is meant to be.

The second openness pitfall occurs when you and your partner start probing into each other's past sex lives. It's natural to be curious, and often we imagine we really do want to know not only the

> 66 The bottom line is that there is no replacement for honesty in a relationship, sexually or otherwise. 99

number of lovers a partner has had, but also just how passionate these experiences have been. However, as a rule, I recommend that you don't probe more into your partner's past than necessary. It is fair—and necessary—to talk about whether you have practiced safe sex, and if you have ever been exposed to or tested for STDs. It is also valuable to share lessons you've learned about yourself and love from your past relationships, and how these have helped you mature into a stronger partner. However, you don't need to share the more intimate, private details. You don't need to know about what position your boyfriend's last girlfriend loved the most, and your partner certainly doesn't need to know about the time you joined the Mile High Club with your ex!

If your partner asks about your past, you can still communicate openly. I'm not suggesting you should lie about your "number" or your past sex life. What I am suggesting is that you explain to your partner why it serves no purpose to go into great detail about specific sexual experiences. In fact, it is a good idea to make an agreement that you will not request each other to share in those ways. The bottom line is that this is information that you will regret knowing down the road. It can be very hard to let go of those images, and they can create insecurities, imagined comparisons, and vivid visual images that serve no purpose. Instead, focus on making your own relationship the best it can be.

TOP 10 WAYS TO STAY CONNECTED

Staying connected to your partner in a long-term relationship takes work, but it is also a lot of fun. The key is to find little things to take joy in that you can turn into a bonding experience. The more you do this, the easier and more natural it will become, and the more you will see your relationship as an exciting, intimate adventure for two.

1 Celebrate small victories.
Don't wait for that big promotion or silver anniversary before you celebrate life's blessings. Instead, celebrate small (or even silly) victories like half-birthdays or the anniversary of the first time you made love. Buy a little gift or open a bottle of champagne and take a bubble bath together.

2 Do kind things without expecting a reward.
Sometimes when we do things for our partner we expect appreciation (and rightfully so). However, you can also occasionally do kind things for your partner without the expectation of reward. Try filling up his gas tank or taking his difficult mother out to lunch.

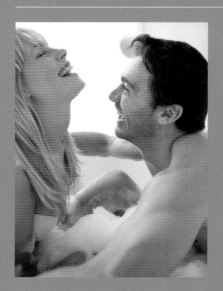 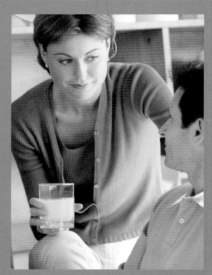

6 Value his opinion.
Women love to vent about their problems, but we often tend to ignore our partner's solution. Show your partner that you appreciate his attention by really listening. You don't necessarily have to take his advice—simply considering it shows that you value his intelligence and input.

7 Plan a sleepover.
Recreate the fun of a sleepover (with an adult twist, of course). Spread out some sleeping bags on the living room floor, watch scary movies together, and play classic boardgames like Twister or Monopoly. Make a rule that the loser has to give the winner a massage (clothes optional)!

3 Write each other love letters.

Emails and texts are efficient, but nothing can replace the written word when it comes to romance. Write him a letter and mail it to your home or to his office. Don't worry about writing the perfect sonnet. Keep it simple and fill the letter with your genuine thoughts.

4 Compliment him when he's not around.

Instead of getting together with your girlfriends and complaining about your partner, create a more positive atmosphere by bragging about his good qualities or talking up his great sense of humor. This will help you notice his endearing characteristics all the more.

5 Be nice to his friends.

Okay, so hosting three loud guys during a football game isn't your idea of fun, but try to make them feel welcome in your home, just as you would want your partner to do for your friends. Knowing that you appreciate this important part of his life is a huge relationship-booster.

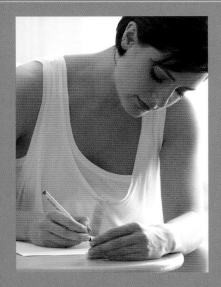
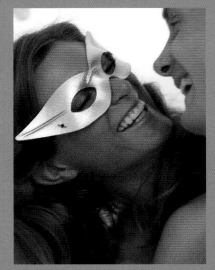
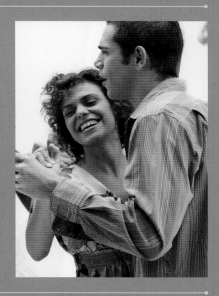

8 Buy tickets to an event he loves.

Is your partner a sports fanatic, or does he love a certain band? Make plans to share this hobby with him. Even if it isn't your style, it will show him that his interests are important to you and that you like to do things purely for his enjoyment.

9 Fulfill a fantasy.

Whether he has a thing for Wonder Woman or is dying to see you in a French maid costume, indulge his fantasy even if you feel a little silly. You might wind up loving your new alter-ego! (Caveat: Never do anything in the bedroom that makes you feel uncomfortable or unhappy).

10 Take your breath away.

Try an activity that gets your heart racing, whether it's kayaking, salsa dancing, or going for a hike in the mountains. If you aren't into physical feats, get your adrenaline going by trying something else new, such as a road trip or a hot air balloon ride.

Ending soft addictions

Intimacy takes work and attention to detail. Every couple knows that obvious interferences like poor communication, an extramarital affair, too much work, too much stress, or substance abuse can take a toll on their relationship. But what about the far more subtle, seemingly innocuous addictions that rule our lives? When people say it's the "little things that matter most" in a relationship, it may be soft addictions they are really talking about.

The comfort of routine

Picture it: A man walks into the house every day after work and can't wait to sink into the sofa for a night of television. He can't destress without it. Is his partner okay with this, or does she feel abandoned and shut out, wishing for some real conversation or a night out? Or, picture a woman who, the minute she is out of her husband's sight, stuffs herself with sweets. The eating is comforting in a way that's too good to give up. It provides a sense of relaxation and even security that she doesn't find in anything else.

Both of the above scenarios are examples of what author and life coach Judith Wright calls "soft addictions." Soft addictions are the seemingly harmless habits that we use to fill the day, to comfort ourselves, and to establish a sense of routine. The truth, however, is that these habits keep us from a better understanding of ourselves, and from better relationships.

In the couples I see, more relationship problems come from the nagging little habits of each partner than from a full-blown crisis. Typically, we write these off as personality quirks, and try to learn to compromise or overlook them. However, Wright emphasizes that we use these diversions to fill a sense of emptiness or to avoid unwanted emotions. Like smoking and drinking, soft addictions take energy away from the rest of our lives. They keep us from focusing on the root of our emptiness and uncomfortable feelings. By extension, they also keep us from being fully honest and fully invested in our relationships. This is why they are dangerous.

Learning to reconnect

Human beings are creatures of habit. We seek out relationships that remind us of our childhood, for better or worse. Similarly, our daily rituals give our life meaning and are generally timeworn habits that may or may not be good for us. The man who plays video games every night or the woman who spends two hours at the gym each morning are feeding their soft addictions in the way that makes sense to them. On the surface, there is nothing wrong with these routines. In many cases, they simply seem like hobbies, and they are part of what makes each person's personality and identity unique. When they become excessive, however, these soft addictions diminish us as people and as partners. They take us away from the real business of life: connecting and loving.

Instead of investing our precious time in soft addictions, we can begin to experience ourselves and our relationships more fully. A good motto for individuals and couples alike is this: Try to identify and face your feelings. Doing this requires time set aside specifically to reflect and share about your thoughts and your emotions. You can't do this if you are spending all of your free time in front of the computer or the television, or at the gym. One way to test if you have soft addictions that are exerting too much power in your life is to ask yourself whether any one routine is critical to your happiness and sense of security. If the answer is yes, then you are probably relying too much on that routine and too little on the people in your life.

In an age of too many obligations and too little quality time, mustering up the courage to overcome some of our soft addictions helps put the focus back on our relationships. Making small changes is where it all starts. Decide to gradually make people, not distractions, your priority. You can do this by putting limits on the time you spend without any human contact or relationship building. When you do this, your intimacy across the board will blossom, particularly with your partner and your children. Overcoming soft addictions is key to your success in life and love.

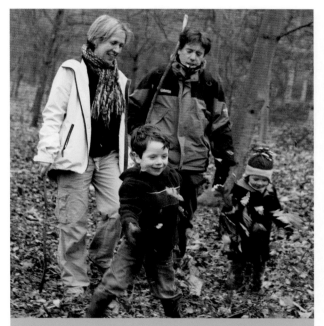

The truth about...

TECHNOLOGY ADDICTION

Two primary soft addictions won't come as a surprise: the television and the computer. Have you ever added up all the time you spend zoning out in front of either or both? In essence, this is wasted time. Imagine what else you could be doing: taking a walk with your partner, playing a boardgame with your kids, actually getting to know your neighbors. To start overcoming the power these machines hold in your life, try having a couple of television-free nights each week. Or, if you feel addicted to email, decide to check it just a few times a day. I promise you that life is more urgent—and rewarding—than any type of technology. (For more tips on how to unplug from your inbox, see pages 182–183.)

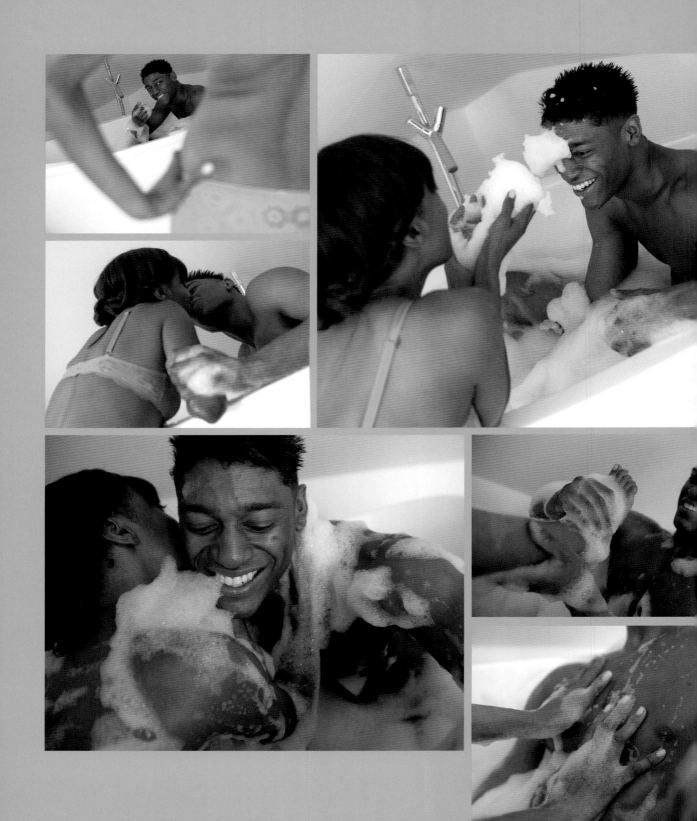

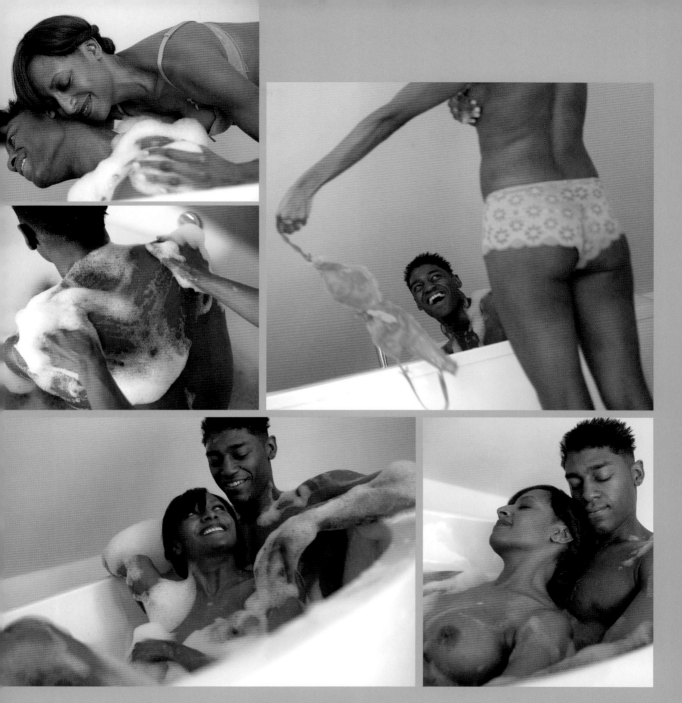

Tub time
For the ultimate in sexy romance, combine a bubble-filled tub with a little bit of striptease and a lot of stroking. Tease your partner by slowly stripping off lacy layers before joining him in a sultry sea of scented water. Use your massage skills to relax and then to arouse, focusing on erogenous zones across his body. Then let him do the same for you, taking time out to playfully blow suds at each other.

The key to love

Hopefully you've learned during the course of reading this book that getting and growing the love you want is a multifaceted process. It isn't as easy as planning a date night or committing to a healthy diet. These things can go a long way in helping to improve your relationship, but as you have seen, the most important changes you can make in your relationship are the ones you make within yourself.

In order to do this, there are two crucial decisions you must make. Firstly, you must decide to take full responsibility for your relationship and your life. Secondly, you must decide to stop blaming your partner or others for everything that goes wrong in your relationship. When you make these choices, you will stop making the same mistakes you have made in the past. I guarantee it.

This new life approach requires plenty of courage and commitment. Like any journey, you might find that you take two steps forward and one step back. This is all part of the process. You are truly relearning how to think, how to communicate, and how to process your emotions. In reading this book, you have discovered new ways to source your true feelings and thoughts, how to shift when you are stuck in a negative place, and how to make gratitude a daily part of your life. All of this will take time and effort to put into place, and you might find that your partner is a little hesitant at first. However, over time, he will see how happy and healthy you have become, and he will want to take part in this commitment to a better life and relationship.

As you make these changes and undergo this transition, remember that your relationship needs to be one of your most important priorities. Taking time to be alone with your partner is key. Equally important is giving your individual self the space to grow and flourish. Without this, you won't have enough energy to fully give or openness to fully receive. Always take time to go to the gym or the spa with your girlfriends, or to paint, dance, write, or engage in whatever creative outlet you enjoy. These are the things that will make you a fulfilled and well-rounded partner.

Doing what you love as a couple and as an individual keeps your relationship strong and happy. If you all you do is work, clean the house, and run errands, you will have a very difficult time enjoying your day or your partner. We all need to spend time simply doing what makes us happy. So, do whatever it takes to make time for the things you love, whether that means finding shortcuts, cutting back on the kids' after-school activities, or ignoring the dirty piles of laundry in favor of watching the sunset with your partner or going to a chick flick with your friends. I guarantee the connection you experience will be more valuable and energizing than any clean hamper of laundry.

In fact, the more you think about what you want out of life, the more you may need to revamp or reconsider your day-to-day schedule. Perhaps you need to step back from the rat race and discover what really fulfills you, whether that is spending more time with your kids, returning to work full-time, or going back to school. Although these choices might feel selfish, they are at the core of your happiness and success, which means that they are good for everyone around you. Rather than being stuck in a negative place or committed to a career you don't enjoy, you will be illustrating to your partner and to your kids that you believe in your dreams, and your energy and optimism will be influential and infectious.

If you are still searching for the right partner, remember that being single does not mean your life should be on hold. Don't wait for Mr. Right before you plan the trip of your dreams or buy that house with the white picket fence. If you can afford it, do it. Travel by yourself or with a group of girlfriends, move to a city you have always wanted to live in, create your own charity, start your own business, find an adventurous hobby, or host a block party in your neighborhood. Do something daring, something that you would never have expected yourself to do. Taking action in this way will help you feel happy and whole, and will also make you more obviously available. Who knows, perhaps the perfect man for you is right up the street. You just have to put yourself out there to find out.

Remember, the only way for you to accomplish your dreams is take risks, take responsibility, and quit looking for someone else to blame. Whether you have been holding a grudge against your last ex, your high school boyfriend, or even your emotionally distant family, the only person your blame is hurting is yourself. In order to step into your own power and create the life of your dreams, you have to take responsibility for getting and growing the love you want. Great love and great happiness are out there, but only you have the key. When you open your eyes and your heart, you will find it.

Appendix A: Mental disorders

Diagnosing a mental disorder is difficult to do, and usually requires professional help. Although I have generally covered these disorders in Chapter 3 of this book, the definitions below will give you more specific information about what each disorder looks like.

Codependency

Codependents Anonymous (CODA) has a useful list of characteristics that describe the codependent. For more information on the impact codependence can have on your relationships, see pages 58–61.

- I have difficulty identifying what I am feeling
- I minimize, alter, or deny how I truly feel
- I feel dedicated to the well-being of others
- I have difficulty making decisions
- The things I think, say, or do are not "good enough"
- I do not ask others to meet my needs or desires
- I compromise my own values to avoid rejection
- I am very sensitive to how others are feeling, and often feel the same
- I believe most other people are incapable of taking care of themselves
- I become resentful when others won't let me help
- I offer others advice without being asked
- I lavish gifts and favors on those I care about
- I use sex to gain approval and acceptance

OCD

If you think you or a loved one may suffer from OCD, consider the list of clinically defined characteristics below. For more on how OCD can impact your relationships, see pages 62–63.

Obsession
- Recurrent and persistent thoughts or impulses that are inappropriate (e.g. not worries about real-life problems), and that cause marked anxiety
- Attempts to suppress the thoughts or impulses, or to neutralize them with another thought or action
- Recognition that the thoughts or impulses are a product of his or her own mind

Compulsion
- Repetitive behaviors or mental acts that you feel driven to perform in response to an obsession
- The behaviors or mental acts are aimed at reducing distress or preventing some dreaded

event or situation; however, these are either not connected in a realistic way with what they are designed to prevent, or are clearly excessive
● The obsessions or compulsions cause marked distress; are time consuming (taking more than one hour per day); or significantly interfere with the person's normal routine, activities, or relationships

Major depressive disorder

The clinically defined characteristics of depression are listed below. For more on how depression impacts relationships, see pages 64–67.
● A depressed mood most of the day, nearly every day, indicated by feelings of sadness or emptiness or by the observations of others (e.g. seems tearful).
● Markedly diminished interest or pleasure in all, or almost all, activities most of the day, nearly every day
● Significant weight loss or weight gain when not dieting (e.g., a change of more than five pounds of body weight in a month)
● Insomnia or hypersomnia nearly every day
● Psychomotor agitation or retardation on most days
● Fatigue or loss of energy nearly every day
● Feelings of worthlessness or excessive or inappropriate guilt nearly every day
● Diminished ability to think or concentrate, or indecisiveness, nearly every day
● Recurrent thoughts of death or suicide or an attempt or specific plan for committing suicide

Anxiety

Below is a list of clinically defined symptoms of anxiety disorders. To learn more about how anxiety can impact relationships, see pages 68–69.

Generalized anxiety disorder

● Excessive anxiety and worry, occurring more days than not for at least six months, about a number of events or activities, such as work or school performance

● Difficulty controlling worry
● Experiencing continued anxiety and worry that are associated with three or more of the following symptoms: restlessness; becoming easily fatigued; difficulty concentrating or mind going blank; irritability; muscle tension; sleep disturbance

Social anxiety disorder

● A persistent fear of one or more social situations in which the person is exposed to unfamiliar people
● Experiencing anxiety or fear of acting in a way that will be embarrassing and humiliating
● Exposure to the feared situation almost invariably provokes anxiety or a panic attack
● Recognition that the fear is unreasonable/excessive

Eating disorders

The clinically defined characteristics of anorexia and bulimia are listed below. For more on how these diseases impact relationships, see pages 70–73.

Anorexia

● Refusal to maintain body weight at or above a minimally normal weight for age and height
● Intense fear of gaining weight or becoming fat
● Undue influence of body weight on self-esteem; or denial of the seriousness of a current low weight
● Amenorrhea, or missing a period for three or more consecutive cycles.

Bulimia

● Binge eating, or eating, in a discrete period of time (e.g., within any two-hour period), an amount of food that is noticeably larger than most people would eat during a similar period of time
● A sense of lack of control over eating
● Recurrent inappropriate behavior in order to prevent weight gain, such as self-induced vomiting; misuse of laxatives, diuretics, enemas, or other medications; fasting; or excessive exercise
● Self-evaluation is unduly influenced by body shape and weight

Appendix B: Lack of desire and arousal

Our sexual lives are prone to ebbs and flows. Even the happiest and most passionate couples will encounter bumps in the road throughout their sexual relationship, including low desire or arousal. In order to survive as a couple and maintain a happy and healthy sex life, you need to be able to navigate these potential pitfalls.

Lack of desire

Research has found that more than 40 percent of women experience low libido at some point in their lives, while around 30 percent of men will similarly suffer. Reasons for low libido vary, but can include stress, hormonal decline, menopause in women, andropause in men, certain medications, and a past history of sexual trauma or abuse, or depression.

Low sexual desire affects at least one in five men. It's the new, closeted sexual issue that no one wants to talk about. Men dealing with low desire often feel embarrassed, since their very masculinity is often tied up in their sexual desire and prowess. Women, too, often feel ashamed or undesirable in the face of low male desire, especially if they have unmet sexual needs of their own. From men's "skirt-chasing" youth to Viagra's new sexual immortality, our culture's messages about the male sex drive are loud and clear: it is insatiable and it is one of the significant impulses that separate men and women. And yet, this stereotype simply isn't true. In the long run, men and women's libidos may be a lot more similar than many of us think.

Like women, men experience low libido because of out-of-balance hormones, certain medications and health conditions, and aging. They may also find their sexual engine sputtering when a relationship is not going smoothly. Call it a sign of the times or a result of our evolution as a species, but men are getting more emotionally wrapped up in the quality of their relationships, and it's affecting their desire for sex.

Low testosterone is the most common physical culprit. In addition to fueling the male sex drive, testosterone increases muscle mass, decreases fat, helps makes bones stronger, and enhances mood. It is man's magic potion. Testosterone often begins declining after age 30. While some men never notice a difference, each year over four million men experience andropause, or the male version of menopause, in which testosterone levels drop sharply. (For more on andropause, see pages 246–247). Depression and certain antidepressant medications can also inhibit testosterone production.

Treating low desire

If you or your partner are experiencing low libido, talk to your doctor about a comprehensive plan for treatment. Lifestyle changes such as committing to exercise and a healthy diet, along with decreasing stress, will have positive effects on your libido as well. However, the most important thing you can do to improve your sex life is to communicate with your partner. Talk about what you are experiencing and have an honest conversation about your needs, whether it is a romantic trip, a visit to the doctor, or a visit to a sex therapist.

For both men and women, Testosterone Replacement Therapy (TRT) is one treatment to consider with your doctor. Many options exist for restoring testosterone, including prescription gels, creams, and patches. Testosterone is FDA approved for men, and is given as an off-label prescription for women. Taking a testosterone supplement and an increase of this hormone can often help improve desire, but it is not without risks. For more on hormone replacement therapy, see pages 250–251.

Another option for men and women is dopamine (a brain chemical that is linked to feelings of pleasure and hormonal processes), which is also being investigated for its possible sexual side benefits.

Higher levels of dopamine in the brain seem to be associated with higher levels of sexual desire and sexual enjoyment. Although dopamine enhancers are suspected to improve sexual desire in men and women, more studies are needed before this research is confirmed. Always talk with your doctor before trying any supplements that aren't FDA approved.

Female-specific treatments

There is currently no medication that is approved by the FDA for treating low libido in women, although one may be on the horizon. Flibanserin, which is manufactured by Boehringer Ingelheim, is a new medication for low desire. Flibanserin was originally created and marketed as an antidepressant; however, it was found to increase sexual desire and "satisfying sexual events" when taken by women who suffered from low libido. It has completed stage-three clinical trials, and now awaits FDA approval (expected to come within the next two years). This would make it the first and only FDA-approved drug for low libido in women.

A recent study also found that Wellbutrin (bupropion hydrochloride) might improve sexual desire in female patients. In the study, one-third of the women who were on the antidepressant experienced improved libido. These women reported fantasizing about sex more often and enjoying sexual activity with renewed interest. However, the authors of the study caution that more research is needed before a conclusive link between Wellbutrin and sexual function can be made.

66 The most important thing you can do to improve your sex life is to communicate with your partner. 99

> **66** Simply put, sex therapy is talk therapy that includes a frank discussion of a couple's sex life. **99**

Lack of arousal in women

Sexual arousal occurs when the body and the mind respond to physical and/or psychological stimulation. In other words, you might become aroused by looking at a revealing photograph of a sexy actor, or you might become aroused when your partner gives you a deep, sensual kiss. Arousal is a key part of your sexual response. When you are aroused through mental or physical stimulation, your body responds almost immediately. Your heartbeat increases, your face flushes, and your genitals become engorged with blood (in men, this means an erection; for women, the clitoris and labia become enlarged). As a result, sensation increases in the genitals, which creates feelings of warmth and tingling in the area. Additionally, the vagina prepares for intercourse by expanding and releasing natural lubrication. These are all key parts of sexual response. Without it, sex would be painful or even impossible.

For women especially, reaching a state of arousal can be difficult. This could be due to lifestyle factors such as stress, inhibitions, or relationship issues, or it could be a result of hormonal imbalances. Whatever the reason, low arousal is something that must be treated in order to protect your relationship. Without treatment, some women completely avoid sexual activity, even though their libido is still intact, because it is painful or simply isn't fun.

Thankfully, there are several easy and safe ways to achieve improved arousal. All of the following options are hormone free, which is important following the landmark Women's Health Initiative study's findings that hormone therapy can greatly impact a woman's risk of developing breast cancer.

Durex Play Utopia: This female enhancement gel was created to increase arousal by bringing more intense sensations to erogenous zones, such as the clitoris and labia. Utopia contains the ingredient L-Arginine, an amino acid that relaxes muscles around blood vessels to increase blood flow and sensation to the female genitals. Simply apply Utopia on your clitoris and genitals before sex in order to maximize sensation and arousal.

Zestra. This all-natural botanical oil is applied to the genitals before foreplay and works to create a tingling sensation. In clinical trials, Zestra was proven to enhance sexual desire, arousal, and orgasm ability. It also works superbly as a lubricant. Many women who used the product also reported that their partner experienced improved sexual satisfaction as a result.

K-Y Intense Female Arousal Gel: This product contains the ingredient niacin, which is a type of vitamin B that helps to enlarge the blood vessels. Niacin can be found in many cholesterol medications, and it is also used in some energy drinks to jolt the body back into action. When you rub niacin on your genitals, many report experiencing the same jolt, which helps to awaken feelings of stimulation and arousal. Like Durex Utopia, K-Y Intense Female Arousal Gel also includes propylene glycol. Propylene glycol creates a warming sensation that can help increase your sexual response.

Ultimately, of course, you can't simply purchase sexual satisfaction. However, products such as these have the potential to increase your arousal, and can help you achieve orgasms more easily and more often. Even more important, seeking out products like these will get you and your partner communicating about your sexual needs, desires, and challenges, which can add up to increased satisfaction and pleasure for both of you.

Sex therapy

If you are rarely having sex with your partner, or if you no longer enjoy sex like you used to, then sex therapy can be a helpful way to rebuild intimacy and ignite new passion. When there has been an emotional and physical breakdown of intimacy between you and your partner that you no longer feel able to manage, a sex therapist can give you the tools you need to repair and heal your relationship.

Rest assured that sex therapy is not strange or creepy or even uncomfortable. At its most effective, sex therapy is a combination of insight-oriented and behavioral therapy. Simply put, it is talk therapy that includes a frank discussion of a couple's sex life (for more on talk therapy, see page 76). The focus is not solely on sex, but sex is a major part of the conversation because it is understood to be an important part of who we are, both as individuals and as partners.

Sex therapy generally consists of sessions where both partners are present and one-on-one sessions, in which each partner discusses his or her needs and personal sexual history. This arrangement helps the therapist discover truths that you may not have shared with each other (or, in some cases, are not even aware of yourself), and find ways to help you share these truths in a safe, open environment. Depending on the issues that you and your partner are working through, sex therapy can last for a few weeks or several months.

Beginning sex therapy

If you feel that your relationship would benefit from sex therapy, it might be a good idea to do some groundwork on your own before bringing it up with your partner. To start, research local therapists that specialize in sex therapy (see Resources, page 251, for ideas on where and how to search, noting that health insurance rarely covers sex therapy because most insurance companies will not cover sexual problems). It is important to find someone who is trained in behavioral techniques and can teach you about sexual logistics and give you homework to do together, and who is also a well-trained individual or couple's therapist. Experience in couple's therapy is especially important if you plan to seek treatment with your partner. It is completely appropriate to talk to a prospective therapist on the phone or in person to get a sense of the therapist's experience, and to decide whether he or she would be a good fit for you and your partner.

Once you have done this, present the idea of sex therapy to your partner in a loving, positive, and honest way. Begin by reassuring him that you love him and want to be with him forever. Then be specific about your concerns. Say that you have noticed that "x" (low libido, lack of variety, etc.) is happening in your sex life and that you want to work on it together. Tell him about the therapist you have been looking at and why you think this person would be a good choice. If he is hesitant, make it about you. Ask if he would be willing to come with you, just for three or four sessions, for your own sake and your own happiness. A good therapist will engage your partner into the therapy during that time, so that he feels comfortable staying on for more than four sessions if necessary.

During this conversation, it is important that you make it clear that you are not blaming your partner for any physical or emotional disconnect in your relationship. Broach sex therapy as a way to improve your relationship rather than "fix" it. This first conversation may not be the appropriate time or place to share any deep, dark secrets or admit that you have been faking orgasms. Rather, it is the first step in creating a safe environment for this type of information exchange in the future.

Appendix C: Menopause and andropause

Menopause, or the period of time when a woman's menstrual cycle comes to an end, is well-known and well-supported in medical communities around the world. Andropause is the similar time in the male sexual cycle when men experience a decline in sexual energy, and has more recently begun to be diagnosed and treated. Both can bring significant changes to your sex lives, but when treated properly and talked about openly, these changes can bring a greater maturity to your relationship.

Defining menopause

Perimenopause, or the stage preceding menopause, begins for some women in their late thirties and occurs when a woman's ovaries begin producing less estrogen, which in turn can cause a woman's entire hormonal system to be thrown off balance. Estrogen levels are typically at their lowest during perimenopause and after menopause. Menopausal women undergo a permanent reduction in estrogen when their ovaries stop functioning.

As you approach and pass through menopause, lower levels of estrogen and testosterone can cause vaginal dryness, as well as less sensation and pain or soreness during intercourse. Changing hormone levels can also cause low libido, low genital sensation, low energy, and a generally lower sense of well-being. Other symptoms of changes in testosterone and estrogen levels include: insomnia, irritability, weight gain, mood swings, irregular periods, incontinence, breast tenderness, and hot flashes.

Sex is often different during menopause, when many women struggle with lower levels of arousal. Lubricant can help protect against vaginal dryness, but the vibrator is truly the menopausal woman's best friend. A vibrator offers a more intense, direct stimulation that can meet changing sexual needs and help with arousal and orgasmic ability. Giving yourself the time and proper stimulation to match your partner's point of arousal is important. If you do this, orgasms may follow more easily.

Treating menopause

Women who believe they are entering menopause or perimenopause may want to receive a full hormonal panel from their doctor. This hormonal panel—which should also test for free circulating and total levels of testosterone—will help you decipher what is occurring inside your body. If you are indeed going through menopause, or even if you are just experiencing a significant drop in hormones, your doctor may recommend HRT, or Hormone Replacement Therapy. HRT can help with sexual side effects and other common symptoms, like hot flashes, insomnia, and mood disturbances. However, it has fallen out of favor recently due to research linking HRT to an increased risk of stroke, heart disease, and breast cancer. This does not mean that HRT is no longer a viable treatment, but it is important that you discuss it at length with your doctor before committing to it.

Prescription and nonprescription medications are also available to women going through menopause. For instance, progesterone, estrogen, and testosterone (all of which are available as a cream, a pill, and sometimes a patch) can help to balance the body's hormones.

Defining andropause

Male menopause is generally called andropause, and it typically affects men in their 40s and 50s. It is caused by a decrease in testosterone. Unlike menopause, andropause can be a very gradual and long-term process. Symptoms are also quite varied and specific to the individual, though common symptoms include low energy, erectile dysfunction, insomnia, depression, hot flashes, increased body fat (particularly in the abdomen), and low sex drive.

Many men also suffer from feelings of depression or inadequacy during andropause. You can help your partner by remaining supportive, and by staying informed about the symptoms and treatments.

Treating andropause

For many men, Testosterone Replacement Therapy (TRT) is a viable treatment option. This treatment includes testosterone injections, creams, gels, patches, or pills, which help to replace the body's depleted hormone levels. TRT is effective for most patients and does not generally have any adverse side effects, although men with prostate cancer should not engage in this therapy because the increase of hormones can sometimes cause the cancer to spread or grow.

Despite the benefits associated with TRT, many men may still be reluctant to use this treatment. For one thing, some men may feel embarrassed, or even emasculated, by the process of adding testosterone to their bodies. Such fears are a natural part of the life-change process; however, take care that any anxiety doesn't prevent you or your man from receiving the best possible care. If you and your partner are interested in exploring TRT to treat andropause, make sure to find a doctor who specializes in sexual medicine.

There are also natural therapies for helping to treat and manage andropause. Men should avoid fatty foods, fried foods, and high-fat dairy products. (Dairy is often full of hormones that can further disrupt a man's testosterone levels.) Herbal remedies such as zinc—which is highly concentrated in semen—are also thought to be beneficial to male sexual health. Regular exercise and prostrate exams are also an important part of staying healthy during this time.

> 66 Giving yourself time and proper stimulation to match your partner's point of arousal is important. 99

Bibliography

Each of the works cited below was referenced in this book, and is an excellent source for more in-depth, comprehensive knowledge about the latest research in sexual and relational health. Use these as resources when you have questions or want to delve more deeply into a topic that resonates with you.

Chapter 1
The blame game

Katie, Byron. *Loving What Is*.
New York: Three Rivers Press, 2003.

Chapter 2
Breaking the pattern

Money, John. *Lovemaps: Clinical Concepts of Sexual/Erotic Health and Pathology, Paraphilia, and Gender Transposition in Childhood, Adolescence, and Maturity*.
New York: Irvington Publishers, 1993.

Straus, Murray A. *Beating the Devil Out of Them: Corporal Punishment in American Children*.
Piscataway: Transaction Publishers, 2001.

Chapter 3
When your mind feels like the enemy

American Psychiatric Association. *Diagnostic and Statistical Manual of the American Psychological Association (DSM-IV-TR)*. Washington, DC: American Psychiatric Association, 2000.

National Organization for Women (NOW) Foundation, 2008. "Fact sheet: Women and Eating Disorders." http://loveyourbody.nowfoundation.org/factsheet_2.html.

UNC School of Medicine, "Survey finds disordered eating behaviors among three out of four American women,"
news release, April 22, 2008.

University of Sussex, "How pop video models prompt poor body image in girls,"
news release, June 1, 2007.

Youngsteadt, Elsa. "The Secret to Happiness? Giving," Science Now, March 20, 2008. http://news.sciencemag.org/sciencenow/2008/03/20-02.html.

Chapter 4
Reconnecting with your body

"High heels 'may improve sex life.'" BBC News, February 4, 2008, http://news.bbc.co.uk/2/hi/health/7225828.stm.

Komisaruk, Barry R., Carlos Beyer-Flores, and Beverly Whipple. *The Science of Orgasm*. Baltimore, MD: The Johns Hopkins University Press, 2006.

National Institute of Arthritis and Musculoskeletal and Skin Diseases. "Questions and Answers About Fibromyalgia," April 2009. http://www.niams.nih.gov/Health_Info/Fibromyalgia/default.asp.

Rutstein, Joel. "Fibromyalgia seems to divide into three distinct groups," *ArthritisCentral,* July 7, 2006.

Wisconsin Department of Health Services. "Wisconsin Diabetes Mellitus Essential Care Guidelines, Emotional and Sexual Health Care," July 12, 2010. http://www.dhs.wisconsin.gov/health/diabetes/PDFs/GL10.pdf.

Chapter 5
Being hard to get

Slotnik, Nancy. *Turn Your Cablight On: Get Your Dream Man in 6 Months or Less*. New York: Gotham Books, 2006.

"Why Face Symmetry is Sexy Across Cultures and Species." ScienceDaily, May 8, 2008. http://www.sciencedaily.com/releases/2008/05/080507083952.htm.

Chapter 6
Unleashing your inner vixen

"Rom-coms 'spoil your love life,'" *BBC News*, December 16, 2008, http://news.bbc.co.uk/2/hi/uk_news/scotland/edinburgh_and_east/7784366.stm.

Chapter 7
Making your relationship matter

Benjamin, Jennifer. "Cheat-proof your marriage." *Women's Health*, January, 15, 2010. http://www.womenshealthmag.com/sex-and-relationships/cheating-in-a-marriage-0.

Breitman, Rachel. "Young women earn more than men in big US cities," *Reuters*, August 3, 2007. http://www.reuters.com/article/idUSN0334472920070803.

Corty, Eric W. and Jenay M. Guardiani. "Canadian and American Sex Therapists' Perceptions of Normal and Abnormal Latencies: How Long Should Intercourse Last?" *The Journal of Sexual Medicine* 5, no. 5 (March 4, 2008).

Gottman, John. *Why Marriages Succeed or Fail*. New York: Simon & Schuster, 1995.

Chapter 8
Juggling family and relationships

Clift, Elayne. "Women's Friendships Lift Moods, Save Lives," *OpEdNews.com*, June 30, 2009, http://www.opednews.com/articles/Women-s-Friendships-Lift-M-by-Elayne-Clift-090629-613.html.

Hoos, Michele. "Choreplay: Housework gets sexy?" *Columbia News Service*, April 29, 2008, http://jscms.jrn.columbia.edu/cns/2008-04-29/hoos-choreplay.html.

Sheraton Hotels and Resorts, "Are PDAs replacing pillow talk? 87% of workplace professionals take their PDA to bed, according to work-life study," news release, September 15, 2008.

"UCLA Researchers Identify Key Biobehavioral Pattern Used by Women to Manage Stress," *ScienceDaily*, May 22, 2000, http://www.sciencedaily.com/releases/2000/05/000522082151.htm.

Chapter 9
Making the life you want

Boser, Ulrich. "We're All Lying Liars: Why People Tell Lies, and Why White Lies Can Be OK," *US News & World Report*, May, 18, 2009, http://health.usnews.com/health-news/family-health/brain-and-behavior/articles/2009/05/18/were-all-lying-liars-why-people-tell-lies-and-why-white-lies-can-be-ok.html.

Wright, Judith. *The Soft Addiction Solution*. New York: Tarcher, 2006.

Resources

A successful relationship depends on wise counsel. Fortunately, there is a wide range of books, websites, and even emergency response centers that serve this very purpose. Use the tools below to help you continue to build your commitment to healthy, happy relationships.

Books and publications

Relationships

The Betrayal Bond: Breaking Free of Exploitive Relationships
by Patrick J. Carnes
(HCI, 1997)

Love Is a Choice: The Definitive Book on Letting Go of Unhealthy Relationships
by Dr. Robert Hemfelt
(Thomas Nelson, 2003)

Women Who Love Too Much: When You Keep Wishing and Hoping He'll Change
by Robin Norwood
(Gallery, 2008)

Mental, Physical, and Emotional Health

100 Questions & Answers About Life After Breast Cancer: Sensuality, Sexuality, Intimacy
by Michael Kyrchman
(Jones and Bartlett, 2010)

Facing Codependence
by Pia Mellody
(Harper & Row, 1989)

Life with Pop: Lessons on Caring for an Aging Parent
by Janis Abrahms Spring Ph.D. & Michael Spring
(Avery, 2009)

The Overwhelmed Woman's Guide to...Caring for Aging Parents
by Julie-Allyson Ieron
(Moody Publishers, 2008)

Self-Care for Caregivers: A Twelve Step Approach
by Pat Samples, Diane Larsen, and Marvin Larsen
(Hazelden Publishing, 2000)

Sexuality for Women and Their Partners
American Cancer Society, 2001
(www.cancer.org)

Stuck in the Middle: Shared Stories And Tips For Caregiving Your Elderly Parents
by Barbara McVicker & Darby McVicker Puglielli
(AuthorHouse, 2008)

Testosterone for Life
by Abraham Morgentahler
(McGraw-Hill, 2008)

The Tough & Tender Caregiver: A Handbook for the Well Spouse
by David Travland Ph.D. and Rhonda Travland
(BookSurge Publishing, 2009)

The Twenty-Third Psalm for Caregivers
by Carmen Leal
(CLW Communications, 2004)

Parenting

Healthy Sleep Habits, Happy Child
by Marc Weissbluth
(Ballantine Books, 2005)

Inspirational/Self-Help

A New Earth
by Eckhart Tolle
(Penguin, 2008)

The Power of Now
by Eckhart Tolle
(New World Library, 2004)

Erotica

Best Women's Erotica 2010
by Violet Blue
(Cleis Press, 2009)

Girls On Top: Explicit Erotica For Women
by Violet Blue
(Cleis Press, 2009)

My Secret Garden: Women's Sexual Fantasies
by Nancy Friday
(Pocket Books, 1998)

Women on Top
by Nancy Friday
(Pocket Books, 1993)

Websites

American Association of Sex Educators Counselors and Therapists
http://aasect.org/
A website where you can find a sex therapist near you.

Codependents Anonymous (CODA)
http://www.coda.org/
Assistance and support in treating codependence.

Griefshare
http://www.griefshare.org
Resources to help navigate the stages of grief, along with a list of local support groups throughout the US and Canada.

Hospice
http://www.hospicenet.org/
Offers support for caregivers, and a directory of local hospices.

National Eating Disorders Association
www.edap.org/
Information on eating disorders and treatment options.

National Vulvodynia Association
http://www.nva.org/
Details causes, treatment, and support groups for vulvodynia.

Office of Research on Women's Health
http://orwh.od.nih.gov
Cutting-edge research on women's health.

Planned Parenthood
http://www.plannedparenthood.org/
A wealth of information on birth control and safer sex practices, as well as a "health center finder" that helps you to find a safe, local place to get tested for STDs.

SexHealthMatters
sexhealthmatters.info
Put in your zip code and find a doctor who specializes in sexual medicine and treatment in your neighborhood.

Hotlines and emergency response

National Domestic Violence Hotline
http://www.ndvh.org/
1.800.799.SAFE (7233)
1.800.787.3224 (TTY)
Anonymous & Confidential Help 24/7

Index

London, New York, Melbourne, Munich, and Delhi

Project Editor Daniel Mills
US Editor Shannon Beatty
Jacket designer Jessica Park
Senior Art Editor Nicola Rodway
Managing Art Editor Glenda Fisher
Managing Editor Penny Warren
Production Editor Joanna Byrne
Creative Technical Support Sonia Charbonnier
Senior Production Controller Man Fai Lau
Art Director Lisa Lanzarini
Publisher Peggy Vance

Produced for DK by
Nichole Morford (Project Editor) and Jo Grey (Designer).

First American Edition, 2011
This edition first published in the United States by
DK Publishing
375 Hudson Street
New York, NY 10014

11 12 13 14 15   10 09 08 07 06 05 04 03 02 01
175350—January 2011

Published in Great Britain by Dorling Kindersley
A catalog record of this book is available from the Library of Congress

ISBN: 978-0-7566-7187-7

DK books are available at special discounts when purchased in bulk for sales promotions, premiums, fund-raising, or educational use. For details, contact: DK Publishing Special Markets, 375 Hudson Street, New York, NY 10014, or SpecialSales@dk.com.

Printed and bound in Singapore by Tien Wah Press

Discover more at **www.dk.com**

It is assumed that couples are monogamous and have been tested for sexually transmitted diseases. Always practice safe and responsible sex, and consult a doctor if you have a condition that might preclude strenuous sexual activity. Challenging intercourse positions might put a strain on your back or other body parts—do not attempt them if you have injuries or ailments and consult your doctor for advice beforehand if you are concerned. Sex in public places should only be undertaken with due consideration of the law and the sensibilities of others. The author and publisher do not accept any responsibility for any injury or ailment caused by following any of the suggestions in this book.

Author Acknowledgments

I couldn't have completed this book without the help of so many people. First of all, I feel such gratitude for Bridget Sharkey, who is tireless and so talented. I don't know how I'd do it all without her. I want to express my deep appreciation for the wisdom and guidance of Jack Skeen and Diana Chapman, whose advice has been invaluable to me personally, as well as to my work. Their advice is laced throughout these chapters. Thank you to Dorling Kindersley, especially Peggy Vance as well as Nichole Morford, who always has the larger perspective and compensates for my brain when it's feeling fried! Thank you to my brilliant agents, Binky Urban and Nick Kahn at ICM Talent. I so appreciate your support and the way you are always thinking and working so tirelessly on my behalf.

A big thank you to everyone at Harpo and the Oprah Winfrey Network (OWN) for making my dreams come true and for giving me a forum to combine all the things I love best. Special thanks to Corny Koehl, Alicia Haywood, Katie Baker and Courtney Cebula at the *Dr. Laura Berman Show* on Oprah Radio. You are master cheerleaders, jugglers, and even contortionists, always smart, flexible, and supportive. The show wouldn't go on without you. Thank you also to Empower Public Relations for your constant attention to getting my voice heard. Also, a big thank you to my managers at ROAR, especially Greg Suess.

To my mom and dad, I love you and thank you for always believing in me and convincing me that people might actually want to hear what I have to say. To my husband, Sam Chapman, thank you for all your creative input, from titling this book to teaching me much of what I've shared here. I also have to give a shout out to my grandma, Teal Friedman, who is a great example of what a powerful, yet soft and loving woman is. She taught my mother who in turn taught me, and I'm hopeful I'm carrying it on half as well. To my three boys, I love you to pieces. One day you'll read this and perhaps understand the women you love just a little better!

DK Acknowledgments

The publisher would like to thank Kat Mead for producing and directing photography, Peter Mallory for producing photography, Enzo Volpe for hair and make-up, Steve Crozier for retouching, Constance Novis for proofreading, and Marie Lorimer for indexing.

The publisher would like to thank the following for their kind permission to reproduce their photographs:
(Key: a-above; b-below/bottom; c-center; l-left; r-right; t-top)
14 Corbis: Jack Hollingsworth / Blend Images. **17 Corbis:** John Lund/Blend Images. **21 Getty Images:** Stockbyte. **22 Science Photo Library:** Ian Hooton. **25 Corbis:** Tomas Rodriguez. **32 Corbis:** Rick Gomez. **35 Getty Images:** Alain Shroder. **36 Getty Images:** Barry Rosenthal. **43 Corbis:** Bernd Vogel. **47 Corbis:** Jose Luis Pelaez, Inc. **52 Corbis:** Rick Gomez (c). **56 Alamy Images:** MBI. **60 Getty Images:** Urs Kuester. **66 Getty Images:** Fabrice Lerouge. **71 Corbis:** Marnie Burkhart. **75 Photolibrary:** A Chederros. **77 Getty Images:** LWA. **81 Getty Images:** George Doyle. **84 Getty Images:** Robin Lynne Gibson. **87 Corbis:** Jose Luis Pelaez Inc. **89 Corbis:** Brigitte Sporrer. **91 Getty Images:** George Doyle. **95 Corbis:** Marie-Reine Mattera. **97 Corbis:** Simon Marcus. **101 Corbis:** Rick Gomez. **103 Corbis:** LWA-Dann Tardif. **104 Corbis:** Oliver Eltinger (bc); David P. Hall (c). **105 Corbis:** Steve Hix/Somos Images. **110 Corbis:** Randy Faris. **113 Getty Images:** Blend Images/PBNJ Productions. **125 Corbis:** Kevin Dodge. **127 Photolibrary:** Photodisc. **129 Corbis:** Don Mason. **131 Getty Images:** Yellow Dog Productions Inc. (cl). **133 Getty Images:** Tetra Images. **141 Getty Images:** E2M Productions. **142 Corbis:** Felix Wirth. **145 Getty Images:** Digital Vision. **172 Getty Images:** Biddiboo. **177 Getty Images:** Lisa Spindler Photography Inc. **184 Corbis:** Richard Schultz (c); David Woods (bc). **Getty Images:** Jupiterimages (bl); LWA (br). **185 Corbis:** Ariel Skelley. **191 Corbis:** Kevin Dodge. **202 Corbis:** Steve Prezant. **206 Corbis:** DreamPictures/Blend Images (bc); Yang Liu (br); David Raymer (c). **Getty Images:** Jupiterimages (cr). **213 Corbis:** Rolf Bruderer. **215 Getty Images:** Cultura / Juice Images. **217 Getty Images:** Jamie Grill. **222 Getty Images:** Image Source. **227 Alamy Images:** Blend Images. **232 Getty Images:** Stephen Derr (r); Fuse (l). **233 Getty Images:** Jon Feingersh (cr)
All other images © Dorling Kindersley
For further information see: www.dkimages.com